The Skin in
Rheumatic Disease

The Skin in Rheumatic Disease

C. R. Lovell

Royal United Hospital
Bath, UK

P. J. Maddison

Royal National Hospital for
Rheumatic Diseases
Bath, UK

G. V. Campion

Hoechst AG
Wiesbaden, FRG

Springer-Science+Business Media, B.V.

First edition 1990

© 1990 C.R. Lovell, P.J. Maddison and G.V. Campion
Originally published by Chapman and Hall in 1990.
Softcover reprint of the hardcover 1st edition 1990

Typeset in 11/12½ Palatino by
Best-set Typesetter Ltd

ISBN 978-0-412-29000-8   ISBN 978-1-4899-2893-1 (eBook)
DOI 10.1007/978-1-4899-2893-1

British Library Cataloguing in Publication Data

Lovell, C.R.
    The skin in rheumatic disease.
    1. Man. Rheumatic diseases. Complications. Skin
disease.
    Skin. Disease. Complications of rheumatic diseases
    I. Title   II. Maddison, P.J.   III. Campion, G.V.
    616.723

**Library of Congress Cataloging-in-Publication Data
available**

Contents

Colour plates appear between pages 70 and 71

Preface   ix

1 The clinical approach to the patient   **1**
     1.1   History   1
     1.2   Examination   2
     1.3   Investigations   5

2 Scleroderma   **8**
     2.1   Morphoea   8
     2.2   Systemic sclerosis   13
     2.3   Eosinophilic fasciitis   26

3 Cutaneous manifestations of lupus erythematosus   **27**
     3.1   Aetiology and pathogenesis   27
     3.2   Histology   29
     3.3   General clinical features   30
     3.4   Discoid LE   30
     3.5   Papular LE   34
     3.6   Subacute cutaneous LE   36
     3.7   Systemic LE   37
     3.8   Neonatal LE   41
     3.9   Diagnosis   41
     3.10   Serology   45
     3.11   Treatment   46
     3.12   Prognosis   47

4 Dermatomyositis and overlap syndromes   **49**
     4.1   Dermatomyositis   49
     4.2   Overlap syndromes   55

5 Vasculitis   **57**
     5.1   Necrotizing vasculitis   58
     5.2   Small vessel vasculitis   63
     5.3   Large vessel arteritis   66

6   **The spondyloarthropathies**   **68**
  6.1   Definition   68
  6.2   Psoriatic arthritis   69
  6.3   Reiter's disease   74
  6.4   Enteropathic arthropathy   78

7   **The skin in rheumatoid arthritis**   **83**
  7.1   Rheumatoid nodules   83
  7.2   Vasculitis   85
  7.3   Cutaneous ulceration   87
  7.4   Joint rupture   88
  7.5   Other cutaneous manifestations   89
  7.6   Septic arthritis   90
  7.7   Management   90

8   **Infections**   **92**
  8.1   Bacterial infections   92
  8.2   Viral infections   100

9   **Miscellaneous disorders affecting skin
    and joints**   **103**
  9.1   Genetic defects of connective tissue
      proteins   103
  9.2   Metabolic disorders   103
  9.3   Inflammatory disorders   111

10 **Cutaneous side-effects of antirheumatic
    therapy**   **123**
  10.1   Non-steroidal anti-inflammatory drugs
      (NSAIDS)   123
  10.2   D-Penicillamine   123
  10.3   Gold   128
  10.4   Corticosteroids   129
  10.5   Cytotoxics   129
  10.6   Salazopyrin (Sulphasalazine)   129
  10.7   Antimalarials   129
  10.8   Allopurinol   131
  10.9   Radiation and other physical forms of
      treatment   131

11 **Common diagnostic problems**   **133**
  11.1   Onycholysis   133
  11.2   Raynaud's phenomenon   133
  11.3   Photosensitivity   136

11.4   Red face and swollen eyes   137
11.5   Mouth ulcers   139
11.6   Nodules   140
11.7   Alopecia   143

Index   145

Preface

The so-called 'connective tissue disorders' hold a particular fascination to both the rheumatologist and the dermatologist, and the diagnosis of, sometimes subtle, changes in the skin can often be difficult.

This book aims to give a succinct account of cutaneous manifestations of the major connective tissue diseases, including the cutaneous side effects of anti-rheumatic therapy, and the main diagnostic and prognostic features and guides to their management. Although the book is intended primarily for dermatologists and rheumatologists, it will also be of value to general physicians and general practitioners.

We would like to express our thanks to our colleagues in the Medical Photography Department at the Royal United Hospital, Bath, especially Tim Browne and Annabel Hancock, and to Hilary Woolf for painstakingly typing the manuscript.

We would like also to thank the following who have generously allowed us to reproduce their clinical and pathological photographs.

Dr T. I. MacLeod (Figs. 2.2, 2.6, 3.1, 5.7, 7.2, 9.20, 11.6(b)); Dr S. O'Loughlin (Figs 3.2(b) and (e)); Dr R. S-H. Tan (Figs 3.4, 11.6(a)); Dr C. T. C. Kennedy (Figs 3.6, 4.1, 6.14); Dr T. Provost (Fig. 3.12(a)); Dr R. Sontheimer (Fig. 3.8(a)); Prof. P.A. Dieppe (Figs 5.6, 9.3, 9.7); Dr S. K. Jones (Fig. 3.12(b)); Dr A. St J. Dixon (Figs 5.9, 7.3(b), 7.8); Dr E. Pascual (Figs 5.8, 8.1(a), 8.8, 9.10); Dr R. D. Thomas (Fig. 8.5); Prof. E. G. Bywaters (Figs 8.1(b), (c) and (d)); Dr J. D. P. Reckless (Figs 9.5, 9.6); Dr R. R. M. Harman (Fig. 8.10); Dr C. M. B. Higgs (Fig. 9.11); Dr N. P. Smith (Plate 4); Mr F. Ring (Plates 9, 10)

Finally, we are most grateful to Lederle Laboratories for
their generous sponsorship of the colour plates.

CRL
PJM
GVC

CHAPTER ONE

The clinical approach to the patient

Most disorders affecting skin and joints can be diagnosed
by pattern recognition based on history and examination
without resorting to complex investigations. It is important to determine the chronological sequence of disease manifestations, such as Raynaud's phenomenon
followed by puffy, stiff fingers in systemic sclerosis and
the eruptions induced by drug treatment in rheumatoid
arthritis. Note also the pattern of disease distribution,
such as the combination of eruption, nail involvement
and asymmetrical arthritis in psoriasis. Clinical examination is generally the best way of assessing the activity
of disease and its response to treatment and it is the only
way of evaluating the degree of functional impairment.

1.1   HISTORY

For the purpose of making a diagnosis it is important
when taking a history to establish the pattern of events
with time and the pattern of distribution of clinical manifestations. It is often helpful to construct a chart of the
condition incorporating the effects of various life events
and treatments. A careful history should include specific
questions about the following.

1.1.1   Skin lesions

Enquire about their length of history and distribution.
Do the lesions itch? Are they painful? What is the duration of individual lesions? Do they vary in colour and
texture? Do they appear individually or in crops? Is there
scaling or blistering? Are there any aggravating or re-
lieving factors?

Enquire about light sensitivity, its duration and pattern

of skin response noting seasonal variations. Are the skin lesions related to episodes of light exposure?

If there is cold sensitivity, establish the presence of Raynaud's phenomenon and its relation to the other clinical features such as digital ulceration. Has there been orogenital ulceration of *recent* onset, remembering that oral aphthous ulcers are common in the general population? A careful drug history should be taken.

1.1.2   The joints

Enquire about pain, stiffness and reduced function which are the most prominent symptoms of joint involvement. Establish the pain pattern: pain due to mechanical factors occurs during joint use. Pain due to inflammation is persistent, shows diurnal variation and is accompanied by prolonged stiffness, particularly in the morning.

Enquire about a family history of skin disease, in particular psoriasis, and joint disease. An occupational history should be taken including present and past occupation. Has the patient been exposed to environmental hazards, eg organic solvents or vibrating tools? Have colleagues at work been affected?

1.2   EXAMINATION

Physical examination should be performed in a room with good natural lighting. The body must be exposed and a torch, or desk lamp, and magnifying glass are useful particularly for examining skin lesions. Since many physical signs are evanescent repeated examinations are essential.

1.2.1   Skin

Note the morphology and distribution of individual lesions. Are they flat, impalpable areas of altered skin colour (macules)? If palpable, what is the size of an individual lesion? (Papules are less than 0.5–1.0 cm in diameter, nodules are larger.) Look for blisters (vesicles are less than 0.5 cm diameter, bullae are larger) and pustules.

Are individual lesions discrete or do they merge to form confluent areas (plaques)? Are they arranged in lines, clusters or whorls? Are they tender? What is their colour (for example, erythematous = red, violaceous = purplish)? Do they blanch on pressure (for example, telangiectases)? Is there a change in skin texture over the lesion? Is there crust or scale, induration or thinning (atrophy) of the skin?

On the face look for the distribution of skin lesions and their relationship to light exposure. A photosensitive eruption spares the chin, the nasolabial folds and behind the ears (Fig. 1.1). Examine the eyelids for oedema and colour changes. Inspect the eyes for signs of iritis and conjunctivitis. Inability to evert the lower eyelid is the earliest sign of facial scleroderma and precedes taut facial skin and perioral furrowing. Look inside the mouth for ulcers, which may be asymptomatic, and for scarring.

Examine the scalp for scarring or diffuse alopecia and for the well-defined, hyperkeratotic plaques of psoriasis. The ears are an important site for discoid lupus and tophi and occasionally rheumatoid nodules.

Examine the nails particularly for features of psoriasis such as pitting, onycholysis and subungual hyperkeratosis. The nailfolds should be examined for erythema and vascular changes which are characteristic of connective tissue diseases. It is easy to examine the nailfold capillaries using an ophthalmoscope after a drop of oil is applied to the cuticle. In a patient with Raynaud's phenomenon, evidence of finger-tip ulceration, finger

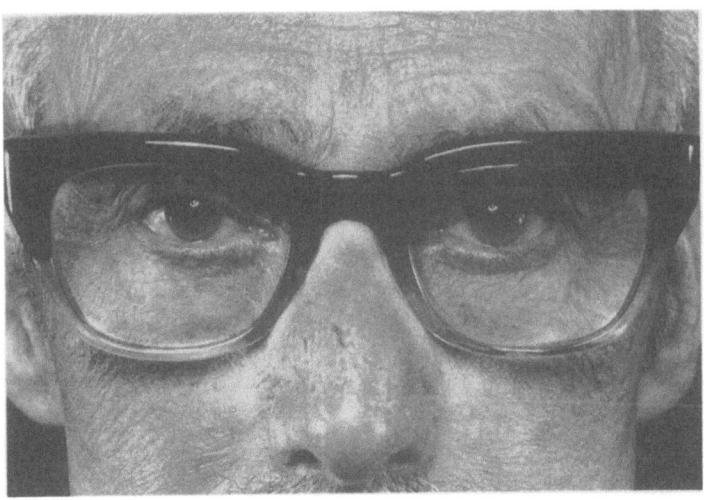

Fig. 1.1 Photosensitive distribution of eruption. Note sparing of areas relatively shaded from sun exposure such as the nasolabial folds and under the spectacles.

pulp atrophy and induration and tethering of the skin strongly suggest systemic sclerosis. Later features of this disease include telangiectasia and calcinosis. The distribution of the erythematous lesions helps to distinguish between dermatomyositis and lupus erythematosus (see Fig. 4.2, p. 51).

The whole body, including the umbilicus, natal cleft and soles, should be examined for the distribution of skin lesions. Look for evidence of balanitis which, like oral ulceration, may be asymptomatic.

1.2.2 Joints

Examination of the musculoskeletal system must include the spine and sacroiliac joints and entheses (bony insertions of tendon, and ligament), such as the insertion of the Achilles tendon as well as the peripheral joints. Muscles and periarticular tissues are nearly always affected secondarily by joint disease but at times they may be the major site of involvement. It is important to ascertain the distribution of disease, the presence of inflammation and the degree of functional impairment.

Joints are examined by inspection, palpation and movement. Cardinal features of joint inflammation are redness and warmth over the joint, tenderness around the joint margin and swelling due to hypertrophy of soft tissues and joint effusion. Red joints are typically found

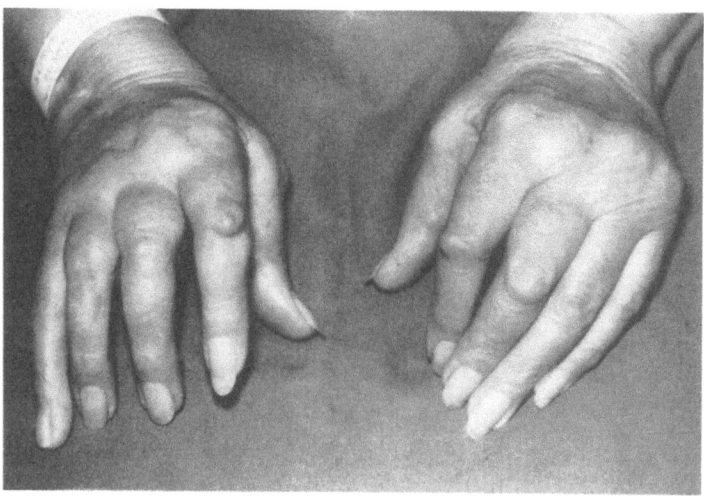

Fig. 1.2 Hands showing typical distribution of joint involvement in rheumatoid arthritis (RA): predominant involvement of proximal interphalangeal and metacarpophalangeal joints with overlying subcutaneous nodules.

in gout, septic arthritis and rheumatic fever and sometimes over inflamed Heberden's nodes. Palpation may
reveal localized periarticular tenderness, for example an
Achilles tendinitis which may be an important clue to
Reiter's disease. 'Sausage digits' in the hands and feet
implying marked inflammation of both joint and periarticular tissues such as tendon sheaths are characteristic
of psoriatic arthritis.

Distribution of joint involvement gives important
diagnostic information. For example, in the hand symmetrical involvement of proximal interphalangeal (PIP),
metacarpophalangeal (MCP) joints and wrists is typical
of rheumatoid disease (Fig. 1.2).

1.3 INVESTIGATIONS

1.3.1 Skin

An ellipse biopsy of a skin lesion is often invaluable if
there is a doubt about the clinical diagnosis. Important
principles are:

1. Choose an early lesion
2. Include the edge of a lesion in the biopsy if possible
3. Include subcutaneous fat in the biopsy (this gives
   more information and allows easier closure of the
   wound)
4. Follow skin folds
5. Avoid excessive forceps trauma by using a skin hook
   or the tip of a needle
6. Mount the biopsy on filter paper to ensure correct
   orientation for the pathologist

A formalin sample is appropriate for routine histology.
Samples for immunofluorescence should be snap-frozen
in liquid nitrogen or transported immediately to the
laboratory on a saline-soaked swab. A punch biopsy is
ideal for the examination of clinically uninvolved skin.
Direct immunofluorescence of the skin is of particular
diagnostic value in subsets of lupus erythematosus (see
Chapter 3).

A Kveim test may be useful in the diagnosis of sarcoidosis. The antigen is injected intradermally at an
identifiable site, near a mole for example, or tattooed

with permanent ink. The site should be biopsied after 4 weeks whether or not a papule has developed.

1.3.2 Investigation of joint disease

A variety of specific biochemical, haematological and serological tests provide diagnostic information or aid the assessment of a rheumatic disease. The non-specific response to inflammation, for example, includes a nor-mochromic, normocytic anaemia associated with a fall in the serum iron ('anaemia of chronic disease') and an acute phase response characterized by elevation of the erythrocyte sedimentation rate (ESR) and plasma viscosity and increased levels of specific acute phase proteins such as C reactive protein. This response can be used to monitor disease activity. The serum uric acid level in suspected gout and the ASO titre in suspected rheumatic fever are other examples.

Serological abnormalities characterize connective tissue diseases and can be used as aids to diagnosis and following disease activity. Examples are shown in Table 1.1. Tests for rheumatoid factor (RF) and antinuclear antibodies (ANA) are important screening tests for rheumatoid arthritis (RA) and systemic lupus erythematosus (SLE) respectively. Tests for antibodies which are highly specific for certain disorders such as antiDNA for SLE can be an invaluable aid to diagnosis. High titres of RF and antiDNA indicate more severe disease in RA and SLE respectively and have some prognostic significance,

Table 1.1 Serological tests used in rheumatic diseases

---

(1) Screening tests
    (a) rheumatoid factor
    (b) ANA
(2) Diagnosis and disease classification
    (a) antiDNA antibodies
    (b) antibodies to RNA binding proteins, for example, Sm
(3) Prognosis
    (a) high titres of RF
    (b) antiDNA antibodies
(4) Disease activity
    (a) complement
    (b) antiDNA antibodies

---

while levels of antiDNA and serum complement can be used to indicate disease activity in SLE.

A plain radiograph is the most useful way of assessing joint damage and its progression. Usually a single view is sufficient and, for example, a single anteroposterior (AP) view of the pelvis with a lateral view of the lumbar or thoracolumbar spine is adequate for most disorders of the sacroiliac joints and the spine. Arthrography, the injection of contrast medium into a joint, is valuable on special occasions, for example suspected joint rupture. Other forms of imaging have a role in specific situations: radioisotope imaging to detect occult joint sepsis and CT scanning or MRI to assess spinal nerve root compression.

Examination of synovial fluid, obtained by joint aspiration, is essential to diagnose crystal-induced synovitis and septic joints. The demonstration of needle-shaped urate crystals demonstrating negative birefringence, for example, confirms the diagnosis of gout. Non-specific features of joint fluid such as its appearance and white cell count can contribute to the diagnosis of joint inflammation.

Tissue biopsies occasionally aid diagnosis. Synovial biopsy, best obtained by direct visualization during arthroscopy, has limited value in diagnosing the cause of arthritis except for rare conditions such as tuberculous synovitis and villonodular synovitis. However, muscle biopsy is helpful in diagnosing polymyositis and vasculitis can be confirmed by muscle, sural nerve or rectal biopsy.

BIBLIOGRAPHY

Burton, J. L. (1985) *Essentials of Dermatology*. Churchill Livingstone, Edinburgh.
Kelly, W. M., Harris, E. D., Ruddy, S. and Sledge C. B. (1989) *Textbook of Rheumatology*. W. B. Saunders, Philadelphia.
Polly, H. F. and Hunder, G. G. (1978) *Physical Examination of the Joints*. W. B. Saunders, Philadelphia.
Rook, A., Wilkinson, D. S., Ebling, F. J. G., Champion, R. H. and Burton, J. L. (1986) *Textbook of Dermatology*, 4th Edn., Blackwell, Oxford.

CHAPTER TWO

Scleroderma

Scleroderma is a physical sign reflecting thickening, induration and tethering of skin to underlying tissue as a result of cutaneous sclerosis. It is the hallmark of morphoea, a primarily cutaneous disease, and of systemic sclerosis. It can also be a feature of other disorders.

2.1 MORPHOEA

Primarily cutaneous, this disorder evolves through a sequence of inflammation, sclerosis and atrophy. The process can involve any level of the dermis and subcutaneous tissue, and either sclerosis or atrophy may predominate in the clinical presentation (Figs 2.1 and 2.2). The aetiology is unknown; an autoimmune basis has been suggested and morphoea-like lesions occur in graft-versus-host (GVH) disease following bone marrow transplantation. Individual lesions may be provoked by trauma.

2.1.1 Plaque morphoea

In plaque morphoea (Fig. 2.3) lesions are typically found on the trunk. Circumscribed indurated areas of shiny, ivory sclerosis are often surrounded by a violaceous margin. The surrounding skin is normal. Rarely, there may be predominant involvement of subcutaneous tissues and fascia (deep morphoea). Morphoea occurs at any age including in children, but chiefly in middle-aged women. Plaques are generally asymptomatic but may be pruritic, or present with a feeling of tightness. These lesions usually resolve completely after a few years without residual scarring although, in younger patients, atrophy may result.

2.1.2 Generalized morphoea

This is much less common and can be difficult to distinguish from diffuse systemic sclerosis. Distinguishing

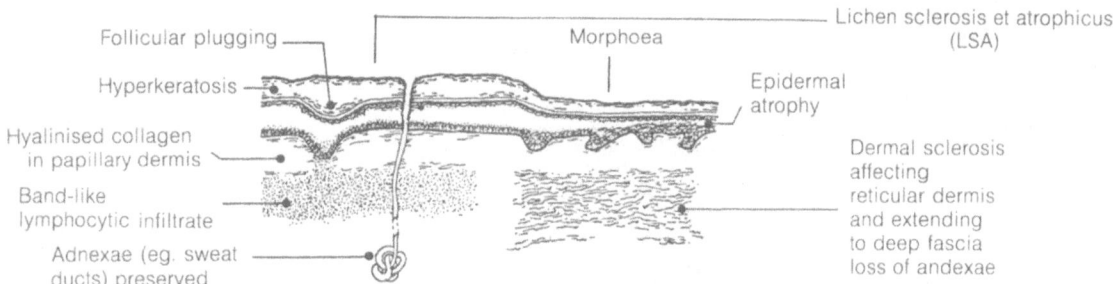

Follicular plugging

Hyperkeratosis

Hyalinised collagen in papillary dermis

Band-like lymphocytic infiltrate

Adnexae (eg. sweat ducts) preserved

Morphoea

Lichen sclerosis et atrophicus (LSA)

Epidermal atrophy

Dermal sclerosis affecting reticular dermis and extending to deep fascia loss of andexae

Fig. 2.1 Diagram of the level of involvement in morphoea and lichen sclerosis. In morphoea, sclerosis involves the reticular dermis and may extend to subcutaneous fat and even fascia; adnexal structures, such as sweat glands, are obliterated. In lichen sclerosus et atrophicus the process is more superficial predominantly affecting the papillary dermis with associated epidermal atrophy.

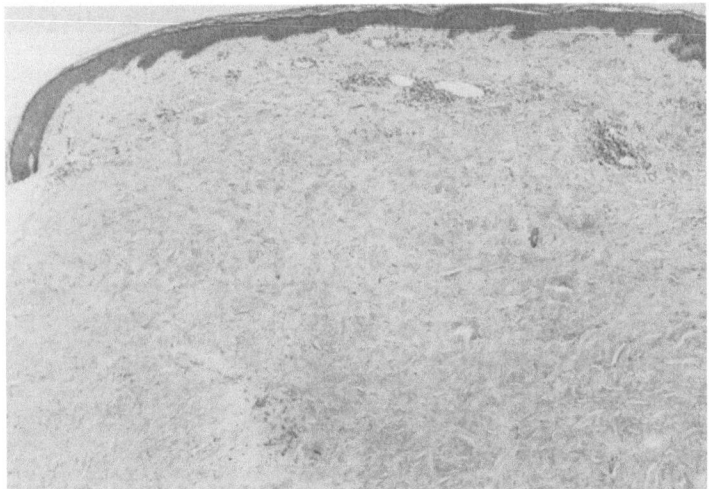

Fig. 2.2 Histology of a morphoea plaque. There is increased dermal thickness with sclerosis of dermal collagen and obliteration of adnexal structures (courtesy of Dr T. I. Macleod).

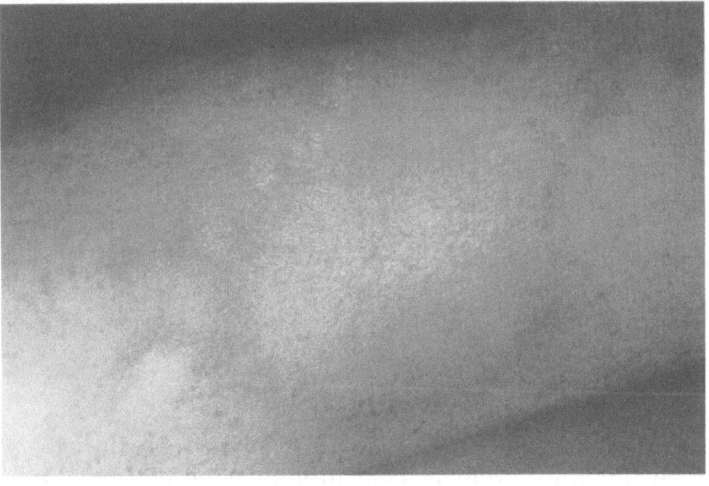

Fig. 2.3 Morphoea plaque: note the shiny sclerotic lesions with an inflammatory margin.

Fig. 2.4 Generalized morphoea sparing areolae; the margins of the eruption are less well-defined.

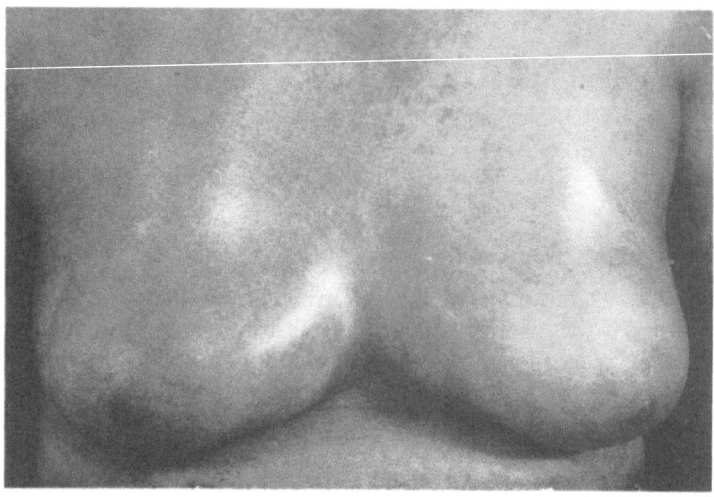

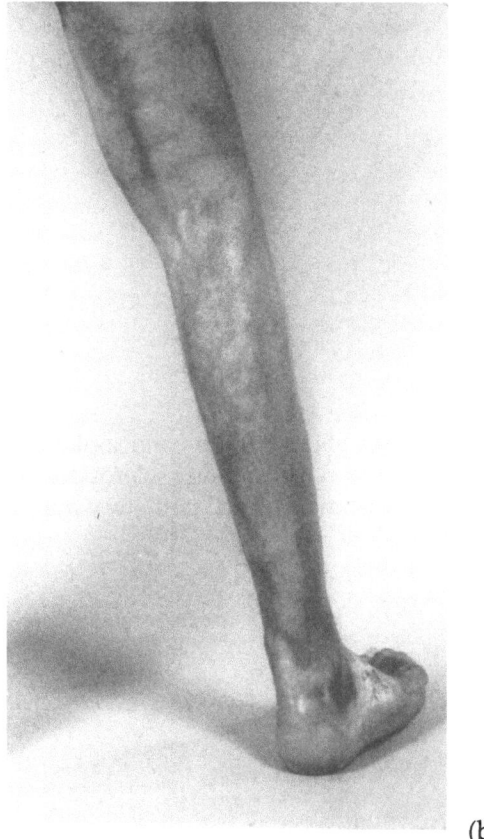

(a)

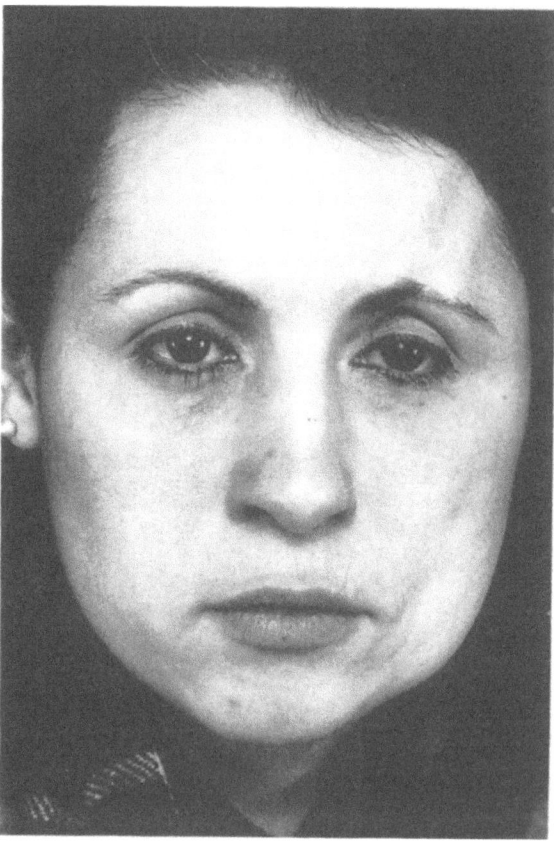

(b)

Fig. 2.5 (a) Linear scleroderma of the leg; note band-like sclerosis. (b) Coup de sabre (facial morphoea) lesion. Lesions tend to be asymmetrical. Note the hemiatrophy in the left frontal area ('en coup de sabre').

features include: predominant truncal distribution but sparing of the areolae (Fig. 2.4); violaceous margin (if present); absence of systemic features such as Raynaud's phenomenon. Affected children may develop joint contractures.

2.1.3 Linear morphoea (linear localized scleroderma)

This predominantly occurs in childhood, but may occur in adults. There may be coexistent plaque morphoea. Occurring chiefly on the limbs and head and neck in a radicular distribution (Fig. 2.5), the process involves subcutaneous tissue including muscle and even bone. Lesions are disfiguring and often painful. Involvement of joints can lead to contracture. Eventually deforming atrophy can occur, especially in children.

Rarer manifestations are bullous, subcutaneous and guttate morphoea.

Morphoea is clinically distinct from systemic sclerosis, although there are rare reports of the two conditions

Table 2.1 Causes of scleroderma

Morphoea	Plaque morphoea
	Generalized morphoea
	Linear scleroderma
	Deep morphoea
Systemic sclerosis	Truncal
	Diffuse
	Acrosclerosis
	CREST
Scleroderma variants	Overlap syndromes
	Occupational scleroderma
	Eosinophilic fasciitis
Miscellaneous disorders	Graft-versus-host (GVH) disease
	Silicone implants
	Lipodermatosclerosis
	Diabetic cheiroarthropathy
	Camptodactyly
	Scurvy
	Porphyria cutanea tarda
	Phenylketonuria
	Premature ageing syndromes

Fig. 2.6 Lichen sclerosus et atrophicus associated with morphoea on the trunk. (a) Clinical appearance. Note the wrinkled atrophic area of lichen sclerosus adjoining areas of ivory-white sclerosis typical of morphoea. (b) Histology showing gradation from typical morphoea to lichen sclerosus et atrophicus. Hyaline sclerosis is seen in the 'Grenz zone' of the superficial dermis on the left of the figure, the underlying tissue being normal. These changes are typical of lichen sclerosus. However, to the right of the figure more typical changes of morphoea are seen. (Courtesy of Dr T. I. Macleod).

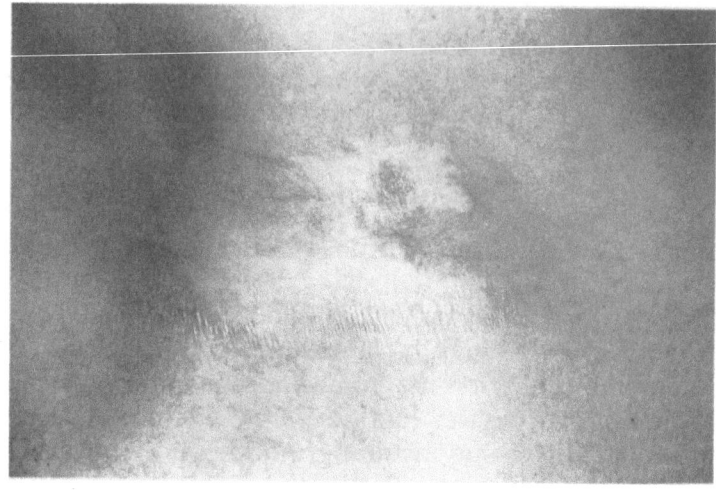

(a)

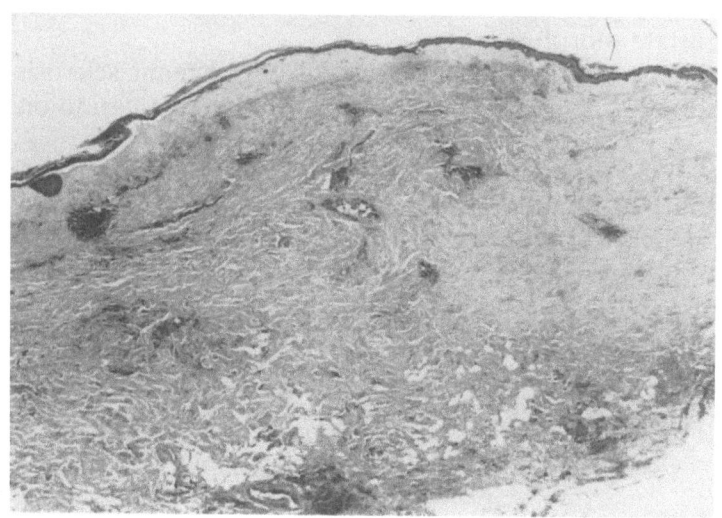

(b)

coexisting. However, arthralgia and sometimes frank arthritis can accompany generalized and linear morphoea. There is a strong association with lichen sclerosus et atrophicus. Here, fibrosis occurs in the superficial (papillary) dermis. This results in white wrinkled atrophic lesions typically found in the anogenital region but also occurring on the trunk and limbs (Fig. 2.6).

2.1.4 Treatment

Plaque morphoea is self-limiting and often reassurance alone is sufficient. Steroids, either topically or intra-lesionally, have been used but may cause atrophy. In generalized morphoea, there are anecdotal reports that drugs such as penicillamine, salazopyrin and phenytoin are helpful. In linear morphoea, physiotherapy may minimize joint contractures and in severe cases reconstructive surgery may be required.

2.2 SYSTEMIC SCLEROSIS

Systemic sclerosis is a generalized disorder of connective tissue predominantly affecting women in the fourth to fifth decade. It results in diffuse fibrosis of the dermis, subdermal tissues and certain internal organs, notably the gastrointestinal tract, heart, lung and kidney. The aetiology is unknown. Fibrosis of the skin and internal organs results from overproduction of collagen by fibro-blasts. Whether or not fibroblasts in affected individuals have an inherent abnormality in regulating collagen synthesis is not known. In early stages of fibrosis collagen contains labile cross-links consistent with newly formed collagen but its composition is otherwise identical to normal collagen. Furthermore all connective tissue components are present in increased amounts in affected tissue. Endothelial cell injury is a prominent feature of the disease and is considered by some to be the primary event. Subsequent production of growth factors from endothelial cells and platelets, such as platelet derived growth factor, and transferring growth factor β (TGFβ) could then be responsible for fibrosis.

Immunopathogenic mechanisms may be operating. Antinuclear antibodies can be detected in over 90% and, in particular, antibodies to nucleic acid binding proteins such as topoisomerase 1 (Scl-70), nucleolar associated proteins, such as RNA polymerase 1, and kinetochore associated proteins (anticentromere antibodies), are highly characteristic of systemic sclerosis and high levels of circulating immune complexes have been associated with disease activity.

Systemic sclerosis-like disorders have been induced by response to toxins (Table 2.2). The major examples are exposure to contaminated rapeseed oil and to vinyl

Table 2.2   Industrial chemicals causing scleroderma-like syndromes

---

Silicosis (coal miners, quarrymen, sandblasters)
Vinyl chloride acro-osteolysis (reactor cleaners)
Organic solvents, such as trichlorethylene and
    perchlorethylene (dry-cleaners, metal cleaners)
Epoxy resins (assembly workers)
Pesticides, for example, DDT (cause Raynaud's
    phenomenon)

---

chloride. A proportion of patients who developed Spanish oil disease in 1981 after ingesting contaminated rapeseed oil showed chronic progression with the development of scleroderma-like changes affecting the face and limbs. Some developed pulmonary fibrosis and pulmonary hypertension. The toxic contaminant is not known, but it is suggested that it might include acetanilide which reacts with fatty acids to produce toxic oleoanilides. Similarly, a proportion of workers exposed to vinyl chloride monomer during polyvinyl chloride (PVC) production developed a syndrome characterized by sclerotic changes in the skin, Raynaud's phenomenon, clubbing of the fingers and osteolysis of the distal phalanges. Some cases developed thrombocytopenia, portal fibrosis with impaired hepatic function and pulmonary fibrosis. Neither of these syndromes is associated with the striking serological abnormalities that characterize systemic sclerosis but vinyl chloride disease has interesting associations with certain HLA-DR genes in the MHC. HLA DR5 appears to be linked to susceptibility. It was found to be present in increased frequency in the affected individuals but more importantly all but one with DR5 exposed to vinyl chloride developed the disease. HLA DR3 on the other hand was associated with severity.

Systemic sclerosis encompasses a wide spectrum of clinical involvement. Cutaneous manifestations are an early feature and the degree of skin involvement often reflects the extent of systemic disease. The histology is similar to morphoea but the process is diffuse rather than circumscribed. It usually starts in the extremities spreading proximally. Rarely, it starts on the trunk. The

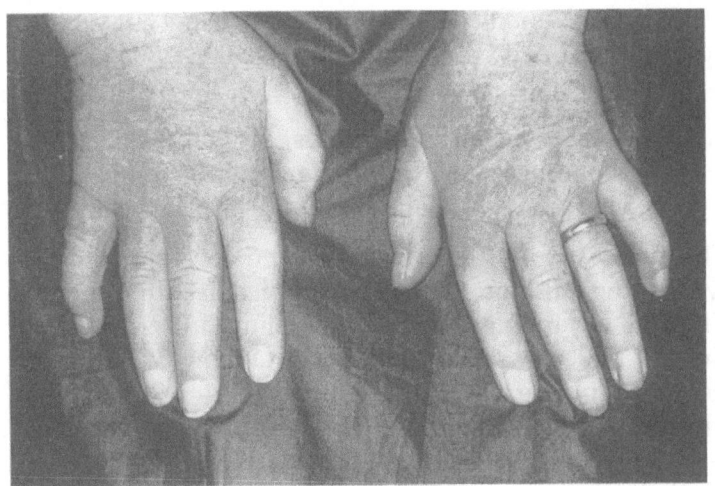

(a)

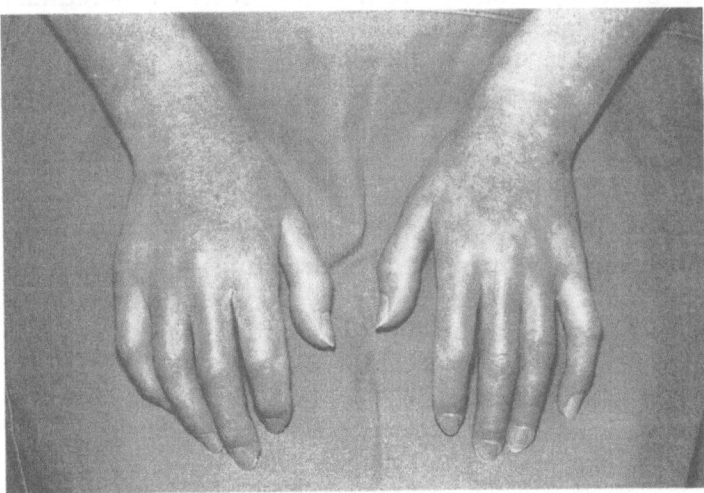

(b)

Fig. 2.7 The evolution of cutaneous involvement in systemic sclerosis. (a) Early inflammatory phase, predominantly swollen, oedematous digits. (b) Sclerosis: ivory-white shiny digits.

extent of skin involvement provides a basis for clinical subsets which have different prognoses. These range from the CREST syndrome with involvement confined to the digits (sclerodactyly) (see section 2.1.1) to diffuse scleroderma.

Early skin disease often has an inflammatory component with oedema, pruritus and hyperpigmentation. Generally, there is a history of Raynaud's phenomenon. Subsequently, sclerosis leads to induration and tethering of skin, and finally after many years there may be involution and even atrophy (Fig. 2.7).

2.2.1 CREST variant (*C*alcinosis, *R*aynaud's phenomenon, O*E*sophageal involvement, *S*clerodactyly, *T*elangiectasia)

The typical patient is a middle-aged to elderly female with longstanding Raynaud's, which is often severe. There is a variable degree of swelling and sclerosis of fingers and toes (Fig. 2.8). Subcutaneous calcification develops in the distal extremities (Fig. 2.9) and may ulcerate through the skin. This contrasts with diffuse calcinosis typical of childhood myositis (see Chapter 4.1). Matt telangiectases are prominent over the malar region, mucous membranes and palms (Fig. 2.10) and are indistinguishable from those seen in hereditary haemorrhagic telangiectasia. They may also ulcerate. A symmetrical arthritis of small joints often occurs, particularly early in the course of the disease, and is sometimes confused with rheumatoid arthritis. Oesophageal dysmotility produces reflux oesophagitis and dysphagia (Fig. 2.11). Sometimes significant pulmonary hypertension ultimately develops, but otherwise major involvement of heart, lungs and kidneys is rare. Anticentromere antibody (ACA) is a serological marker for this group (Fig. 2.12). It is present in up to

Fig. 2.8 Sclerodactyly and digital ulceration in a patient with CREST.

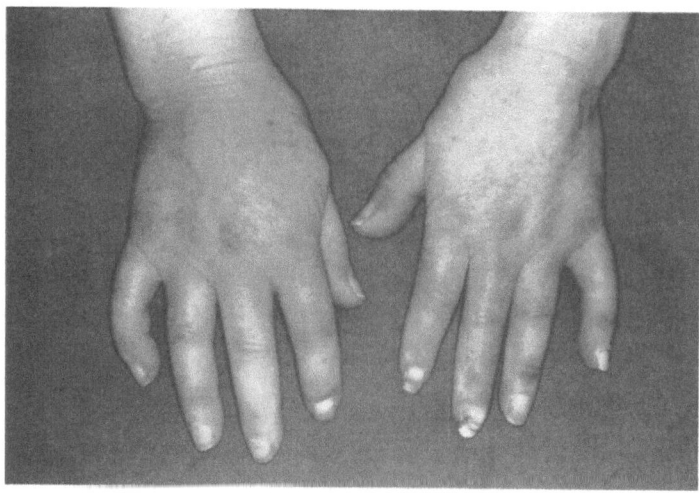

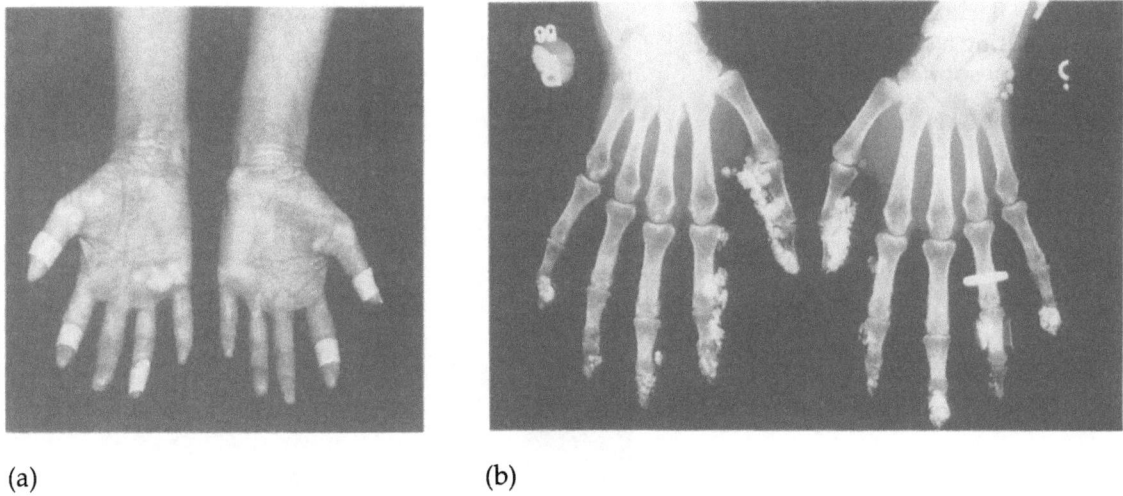

(a)   (b)

Fig. 2.9 Calcinosis of digits. (a) Calcific nodules typically found on the fingers. (b) The radiograph confirms calcification.

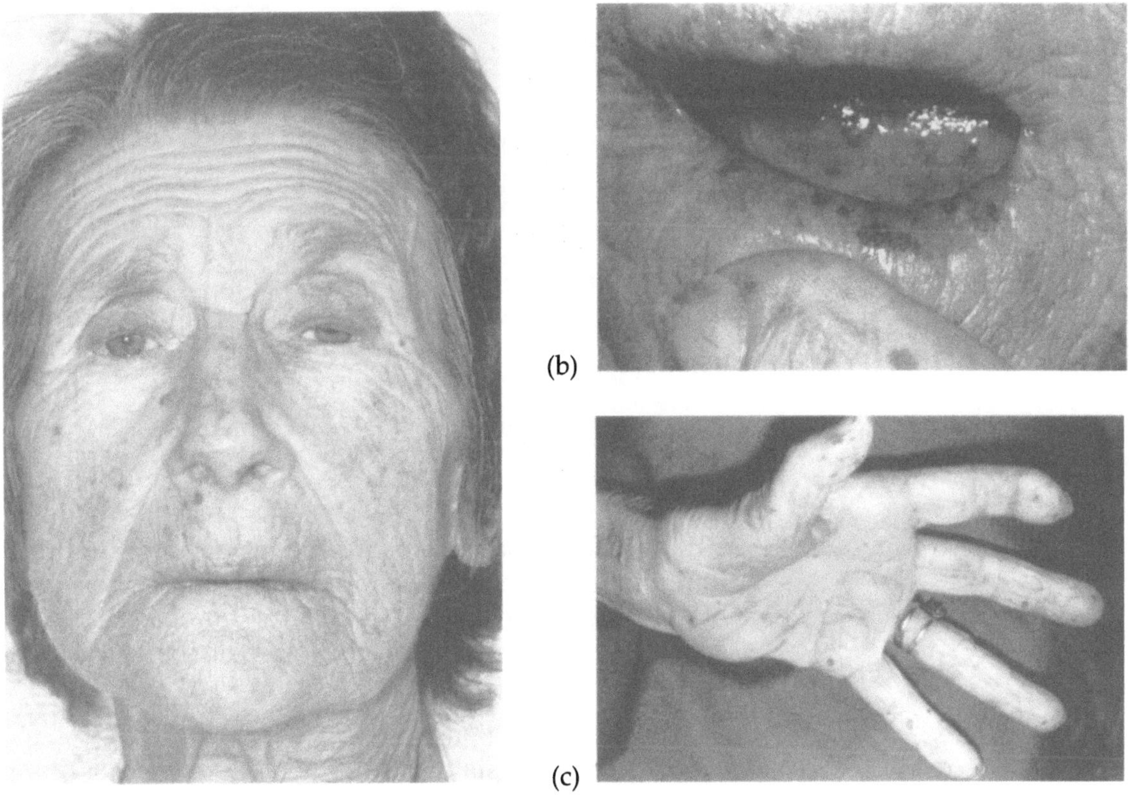

(a)   (b)   (c)

Fig. 2.10 Matt telangiectasia of (a) face, (b) lips and fingers, (c) palms.

Fig. 2.11 Barium swallow demonstrating a dilated hypotonic oesophagus.

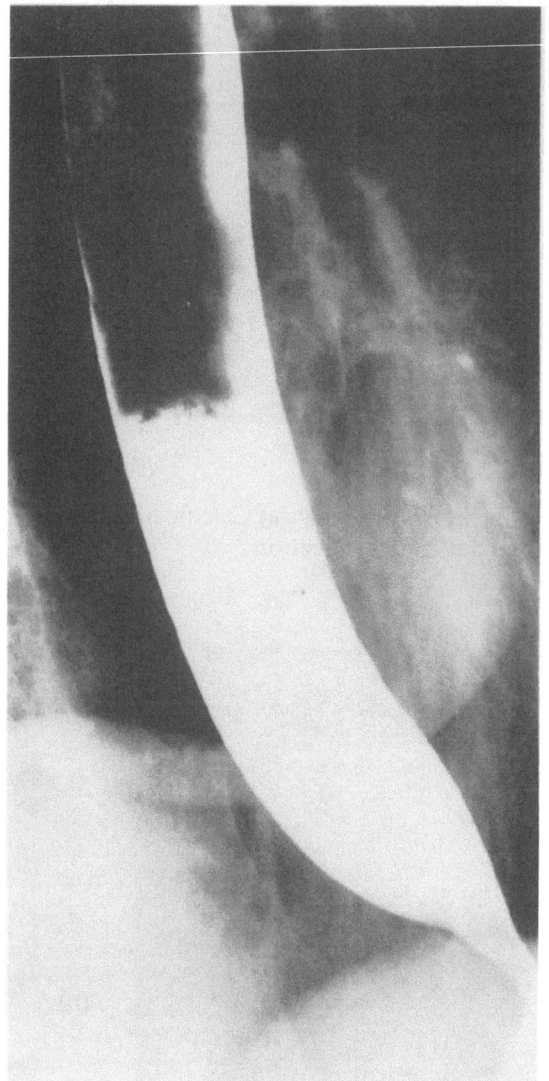

90% of CREST patients using the technique of indirect immunofluorescence with rapidly growing monolayers of cell lines such as Hep-2 cells or fibroblasts as the substrate. Primary biliary cirrhosis can be associated with the CREST variant.

2.2.2 Acrosclerosis

This implies cutaneous involvement of the extremities. In addition to the distal forearms, hands, lower legs and

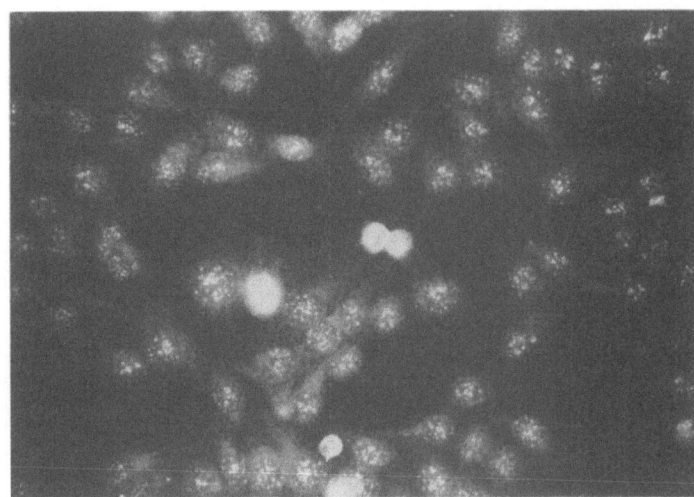

Fig. 2.12 Indirect immunofluorescence on Hep-2 cells showing an ACA pattern with discrete speckles in interphase nuclei which collect on the metaphase plate during cell division.

feet, affected sites include the perioral and periorbital skin and the neck. Like CREST it occurs characteristically in middle-aged women, it is slowly progressive and Raynaud's is prominent. However, sclerosis is more marked and morbidity is greater than in CREST. Cutaneous and periarticular sclerosis lead to progressive contracture of the fingers (Fig. 2.13). Ischaemic ulcers may occur on the finger tips or knuckles (Fig. 2.14). Chronic paronychia is common and superficial gangrene may occur (Fig. 2.15). The fingers are tapered with pulp

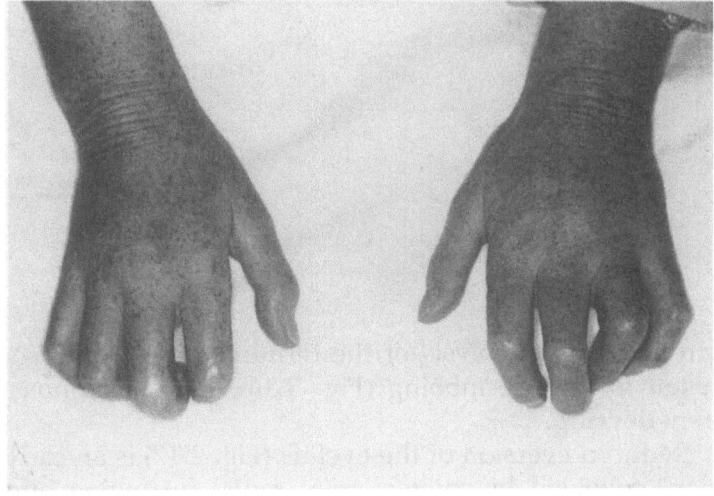

Fig. 2.13 Contracture of the fingers in acrosclerosis.

Fig. 2.14 Ischaemic ulcers on finger tips.

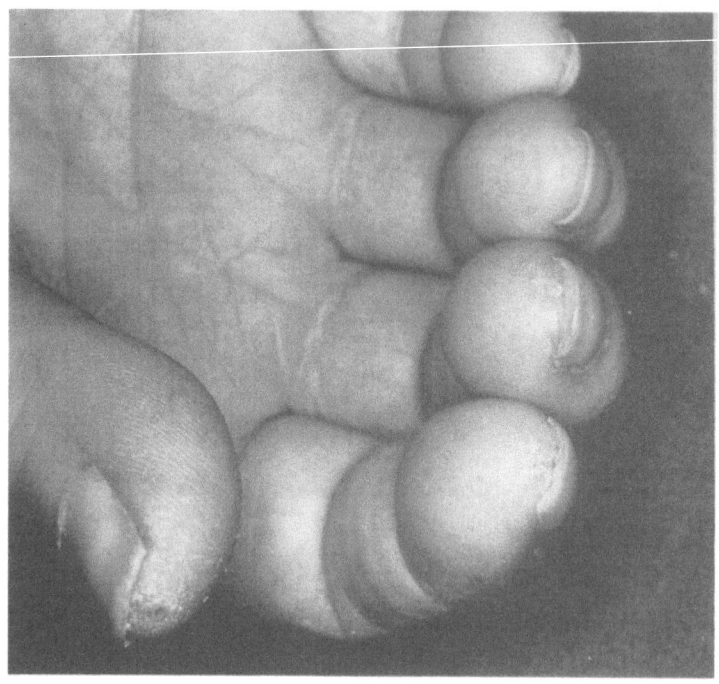

Fig. 2.15 Chronic paronychia in acrosclerosis.

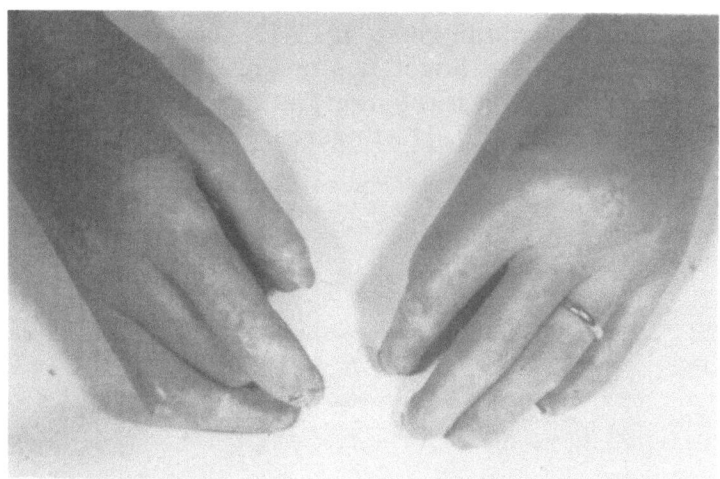

atrophy and osteolysis of the terminal phalanges may result in pseudoclubbing (Fig. 2.16). Later, calcinosis may develop.

Reduced eversion of the eyelids (Fig. 2.17) is an early sign, followed by microstomia, radial furrowing and

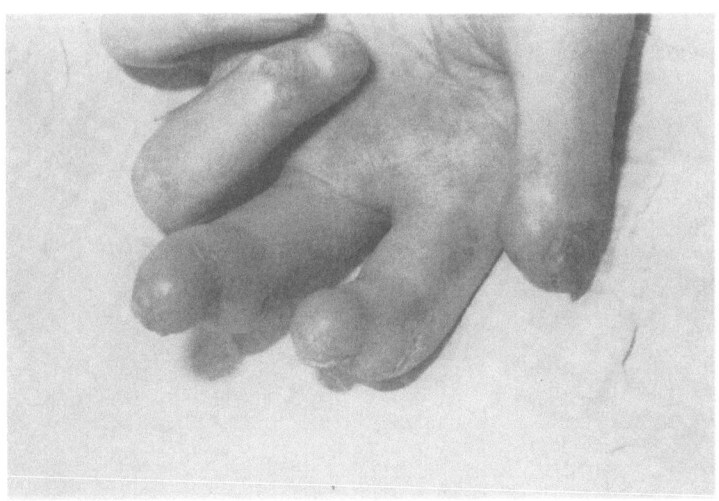

Fig. 2.16 Pulp atrophy and pseudoclubbing.

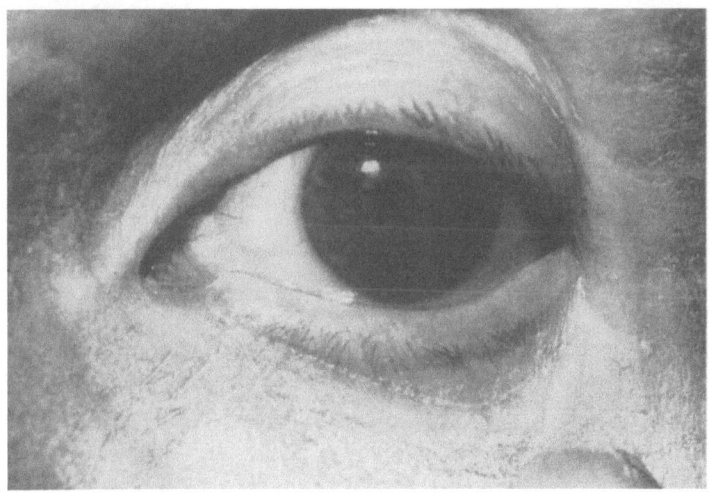

Fig. 2.17 Reduced eversion of the lower eyelid in acrosclerosis; this is one of the earliest features of facial involvement in systemic sclerosis.

telangiectasia (Fig. 2.18). Mucous membrane involvement, sometimes compounded by Sjögren's syndrome, contributes to poor dental hygiene and problems with swallowing. A polyarthritis predominantly affecting hands, wrists and knees occurs early (Fig. 2.19). A small number develop myositis indistinguishable from primary polymyositis (see Chapter 4). Gastrointestinal involvement, particularly oesophageal dysfunction, is the most important systemic feature.

Diffuse intestinal involvement frequently results in

Fig. 2.18 Facial appearance in acrosclerosis; note radial furrowing of the mouth, matt telangiectasia, pinched nose and loss of skin folds below eyes.

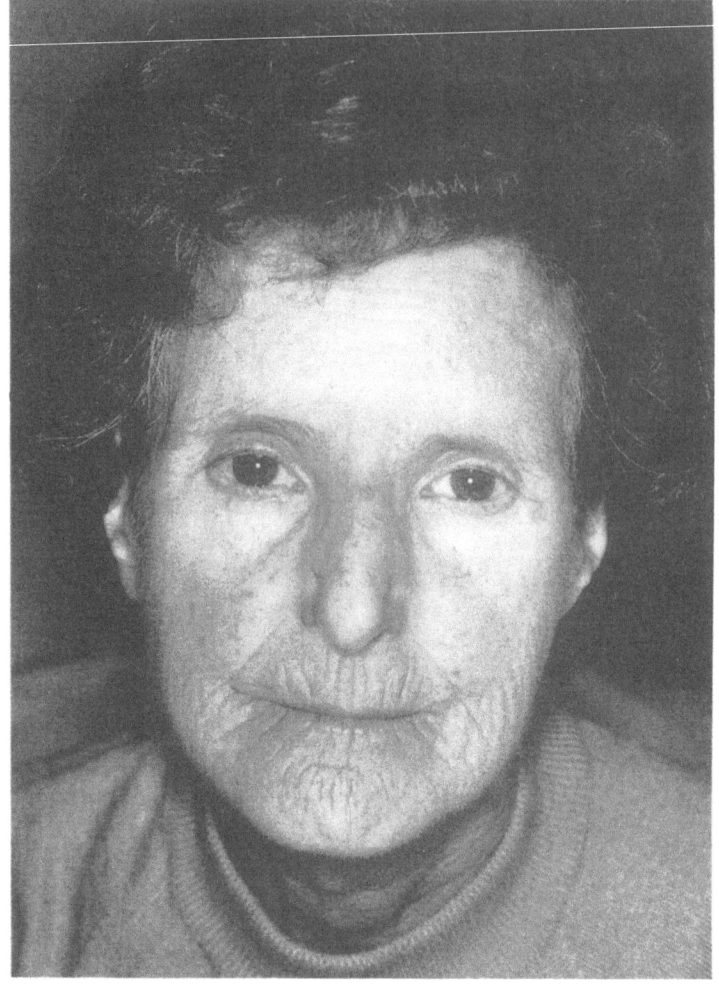

bacterial overgrowth producing symptoms such as abdominal pain and diarrhoea occasionally with frank malabsorption. There is usually pulmonary involvement with intestinal fibrosis but respiratory failure is uncommon. Similarly, significant cardiac and renovascular disease is rare in this group.

2.2.3 Diffuse scleroderma

This is usually more rapidly progressive with sclerosis extending proximally on to the trunk, sometimes encasing the entire body (en cuirasse). In some cases, the

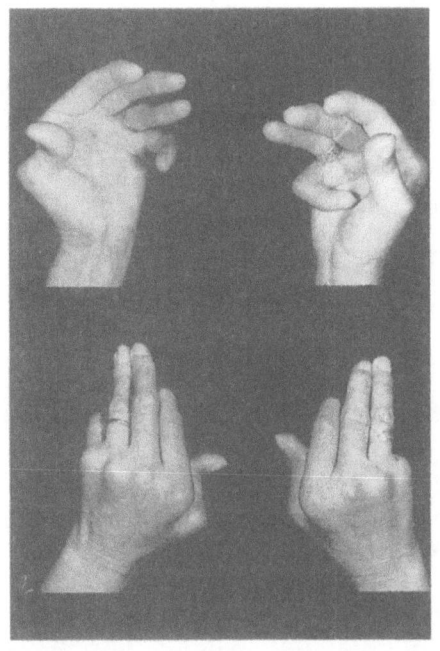

(a)

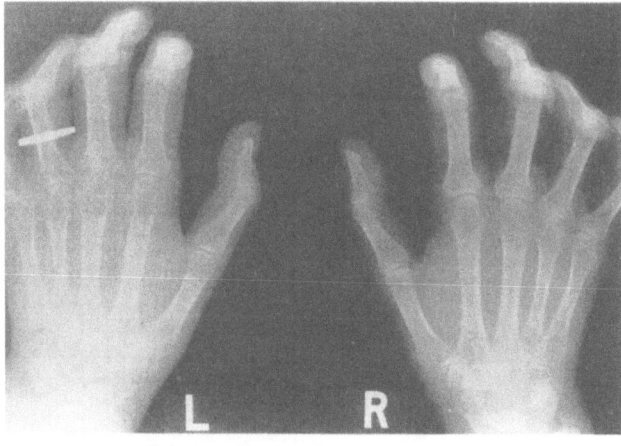

(b)

Fig. 2.19 Joint involvement in systemic sclerosis. (a) Hands showing joint contractures, mostly due to joint capsule and tendon sheath involvement. (b) Radiograph of hands in diffuse scleroderma. Despite joint deformity, erosions are absent.

sclerosis is restricted to the trunk (truncal scleroderma). In early disease inflammatory features are often pronounced. Hyperpigmentation may resemble Addison's disease (Fig. 2.20) although hypopigmentation may be a feature in negroid skin. Raynaud's is not invariably present and calcinosis and telangiectasia are infrequent. Systemic involvement involving the heart, lungs and kidneys is often severe and these patients are at risk of developing highly malignant arterial hypertension leading to rapidly progressive and irreversible renal failure. Although hypertension and high plasma renin levels are the rule, renal failure occasionally occurs with normal blood pressure. As in other patients, polyarthritis may occur, but a striking feature is often a tendinitis accompanied by characteristic coarse crepitus particularly over the flexor and extensor tendons of the wrist. This has been related to collagen deposition on the surfaces of the tendon sheaths and overlying fascia. Anticentromere antibodies are rarely found in these

Fig. 2.20 Hyperpigmentation
in diffuse scleroderma.

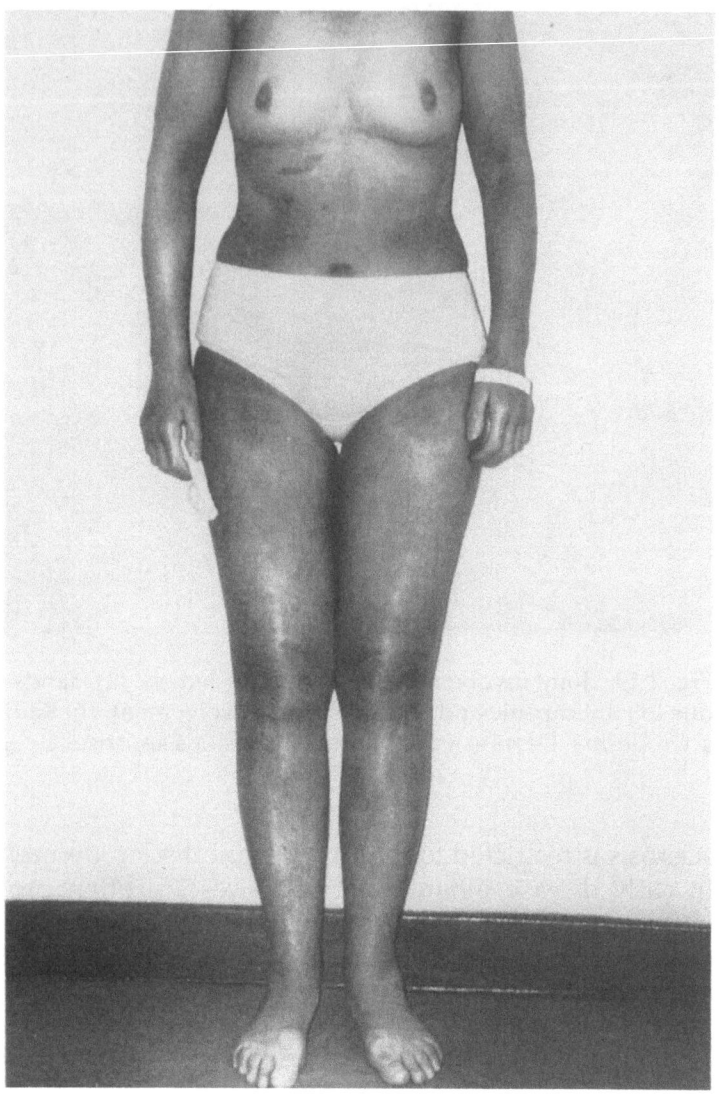

patients, but in approximately one-third antibodies are
directed to topoisomerase 1 (Scl-70).

2.2.4 Differential diagnosis

Early stages of systemic sclerosis may be difficult to
diagnose. Stiff, swollen fingers occur in polyarthritis including rheumatoid arthritis, and induration of truncal
skin is a feature of generalized morphoea (section 2.1.2),

eosinophilic fasciitis (section 2.3) and scleroedema of Buschke. This last condition is often of rapid onset following inoculation or infection, affects primarily the neck, shoulder and upper arms and can be distinguished clinically from scleroderma by wrinkling the overlying skin.

2.2.5 Treatment

This is predominantly symptomatic. The hands and feet should be protected against cold and heated gloves are sometimes helpful. Drug therapy for Raynaud's phenomenon includes the use of calcium channel blockers, alpha receptor antagonists and antifibrinolytic agents. Infusions of vasodilators such as prostaglandin E1 and prostacyclin may be helpful in ischaemic crises. Even if gangrene supervenes, it is usually superficial and does not require radical surgery. Digital ulcers may respond to topical application of nitroglycerine or stable prostaglandins. Emollients are often helpful to prevent dry

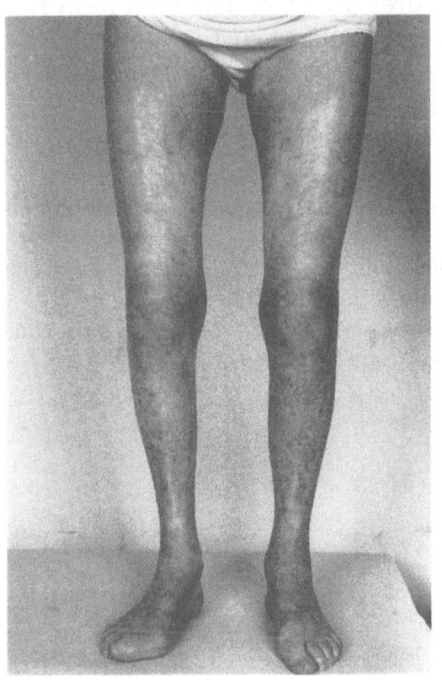

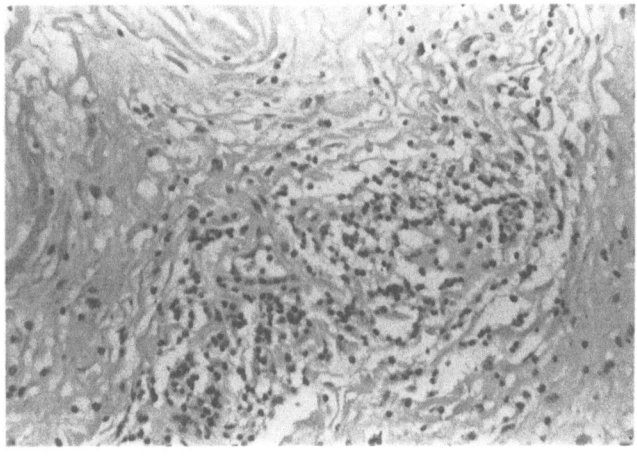

(a)   (b)

Fig. 2.21   Eosinophilic fasciitis. (a) Clinical involvement of legs showing tense induration of the skin. (b) Histological features including eosinophilic infiltration and fibrosis of deep fascia.

skin and pruritus. Facial telangiectasia can be effectively masked by cosmetic camouflage.

Specific therapy is disappointing. D-penicillamine and colchicine may improve cutaneous sclerosis but have little effect on systemic features. Captopril and other angiotensin converting enzyme inhibitors, increasingly used in hypertensive crises, have been reported to reduce skin involvement. The use of systemic corticosteroids is controversial but may benefit early disease.

2.3 EOSINOPHILIC FASCIITIS

The onset is frequently acute and the condition develops typically in young males after extreme exertion. Painful induration affects particularly the proximal limbs (Fig. 2.21a), it may be accompanied by carpal tunnel syndrome but not by Raynaud's phenomenon. A deep biopsy is required to demonstrate the characteristic infiltrate in the deep fascia (Fig. 2.21b). A blood eosinophilia occurs and aplastic anaemia has been reported, but other systemic features are rare. The condition frequently responds to systemic corticosteroids and may be self-limiting.

BIBLIOGRAPHY

Jablonska, S. (1975) *Scleroderma and Pseudoscleroderma*. Polish Medical Publishers, Warsaw.

Jayson, M. I. V. and Black, C. M. (1988) *Systemic Sclerosis: Scleroderma*. John Wiley & Sons, Chichester.

Rodnan, G. P. (1978) Progressive systemic sclerosis, *Immunological Diseases* (ed. Samter, M.), Little Brown & Co., Boston, 1109–41.

CHAPTER THREE

Cutaneous manifestations of lupus erythematosus

Lupus erythematosus (LE) represents a spectrum ranging from localized cutaneous disease, in which cell mediated immunity predominates, to systemic LE with marked serological abnormalities (Table 3.1).

3.1 AETIOLOGY AND PATHOGENESIS

The aetiology is unknown, but it is current thought that lupus is the result of an environmental trigger acting on a genetically susceptible host. Multiple genes appear to be involved and in SLE, for example, this is shown in the marked female preponderance, susceptibility of certain races and association with HLA antigen in the major histocompatibility complex in chromosome six, particularly with Class II antigens such as HLA DR2 and HLA DR3. Environmental factors include ultraviolet

Table 3.1 Spectrum of cutaneous lupus erythematosus (LE)

Chronic cutaneous (discoid) LE	————————	Systemic LE
	Subacute cutaneous	
	LE profundus	
		Acute cutaneous
Cell mediated immunity (T Cell)	————————	Immune complex disease (B Cell)

irradiation. Chronic cutaneous lesions occur generally in light exposed regions. Furthermore, approximately 30% of SLE patients are photosensitive. Ultraviolet irradiation specifically denatures DNA to form thymine dimers which are much more immunogenic than native DNA. There is considerable speculation that some cases of SLE might be precipitated by viral infection.

Retroviruses have come under particular scrutiny following the observation that C-type retrovirus encoded proteins induce an immune response in the NZB/W mouse model of lupus. There were similar findings in humans with SLE with C-type virus related proteins; in some cases these are complexed to antibody in the biopsies of clinically involved skin and kidney. Recent studies, however, have failed to demonstrate serological evidence in epidemiological studies or to isolate specific viral products in tissues of patients. Lupus-like syndromes can be induced by certain drugs. Some of the

Table 3.2   Drug induced lupus

DRUGS KNOWN TO PRECIPITATE SLE		
Frequent association	*Rare association*	
Procainamide	Oral contraceptives	Penicillamine
Hydralazine	Chlorthalidone	Captopril
Isoniazid	Griseofulvin	Prazosin
Anticonvulsants	Levodopa	Propylthiouracil
Chlorpromazine	Methyldopa	Quinidine
	Methysergide	Reserpine
	Penicillin	Streptomycin
		Sulphonamides
		Tetracycline

CLINICAL FEATURES	
Common	*Rare*
Polyarthritis	Renal and neuropsychiatric
Rash	disease
Pleurisy/pericarditis	Antinative DNA
Pulmonary infiltrates	Low serum complement
High titre ANA	
(mainly to histones)	
Resolution when drug stopped	

Table 3.3   Drug induced lupus – risk factors

Sufficient cumulative dose of drug
Slow acetylator status
Older age
Sex (female preponderance)
Presence of HLA DR4 (hydralazine)

Table 3.4   Immunological abnormalities in SLE

A.	Humoral	Hypergammaglobulinaemia
		Autoantibodies to selected cell constituents such as nucleosome: DNA, histones and RNA binding proteins: Sm, U1RNP, Ro, La
		Circulating immune complexes
B.	Cellular	Primary B cell defect
		Loss of 'suppressor' T cells
		Reduced interleukin-2 regulation
		Reduced reticuloendothelial function

implicated drugs and the features of drug-induced lupus are listed in Table 3.2. Drug induced lupus is an excellent example of how an environmental agent interacts with host factors (Table 3.3).

Immunological abnormalities are striking in SLE and are listed in Table 3.4. Autoantibodies directed especially to nuclear constituents are present in virtually all patients, and there is circumstantial evidence that certain antibodies have a direct role in the pathogenesis of tissue lesions. Lupus nephritis, for example, demonstrates features on immunohistology and electron microscopy of an immune complex mediated disease and autoantibodies to DNA have been implicated in this. There is also evidence of autoantibody involvement in other clinical features seen in the disease such as vasculitis, serositis and certain aspects of CNS involvement.

3.2   HISTOLOGY

Histology of the skin reflects the evolution of an individual lesion rather than the overall clinical category of LE (Table 3.5 and Fig. 3.1). The features common to most biopsies of cutaneous lupus are liquefaction de-

Table 3.5 Histological changes in lupus erythematosus

Early features	Later features
Liquefaction degeneration is the unifying feature (see Fig. 3.1)	Hyperkeratosis
Perivascular infiltrate of T lymphocytes	Follicular plugging
Dermal oedema	Epidermal atrophy
	Atrophy of adnexal structures

Immunofluorescence

Granular deposition of immunoglobulins and complement in lesions and sometimes in normal skin (see section 3.9.2)

generation of the dermoepidermal junction and a mononuclear cell infiltrate. This is composed predominantly of T cells with approximately equal numbers of cells carrying the CD4 and CD8 phenotype. Langerhans cells are absent in the lesions and the keratinocytes show striking expression of DR antigens. Changes such as epidermal atrophy and adnexal scarring, hyperkeratosis and follicular plugging are most marked in chronic discoid lesions.

3.3 GENERAL CLINICAL FEATURES

There is a striking female preponderance especially in SLE when the female to male ratio is approximately 9:1. Onset occurs at any age, primarily 20–40. There are racial variations, with increased prevalence of SLE in Afrocaribbeans in America and the Chinese in Malaysia and Hong Kong. There does not seem to be a corresponding increase in SLE in Africa and China which again points to an interplay between environmental and host factors.

3.4 DISCOID LE (DLE)

Typically lesions occur in light exposed areas, particularly the head and neck (including scalp). Lesions are well demarcated, erythematous and hyperkeratotic with follicular plugging, atrophy, telangiectasia and hypopigmentation or hyperpigmentation. They may

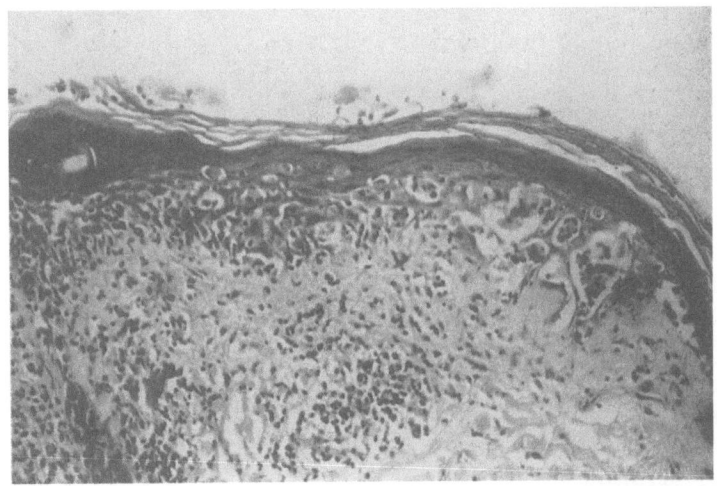

(a)

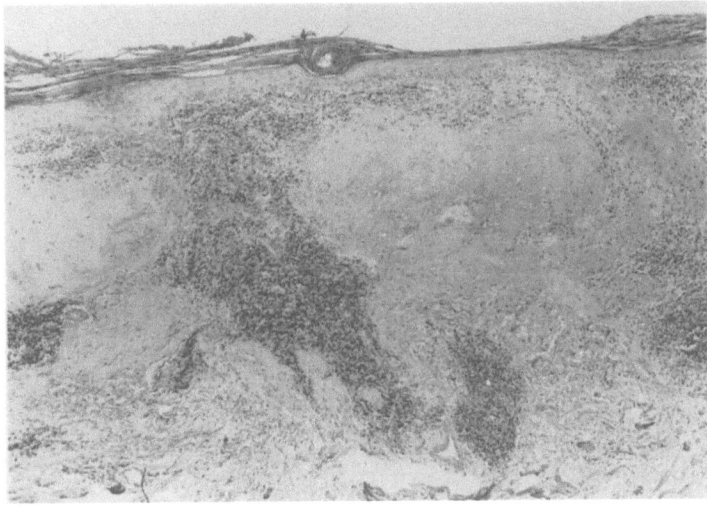

(b)

Fig. 3.1 Histology of LE. (a) Early features including liquefaction degeneration at the dermoepidermal junction, lymphocytic infiltration and dermal oedema. (b) Histology of established plaque of DLE showing hyperkeratosis, follicular plugging, atrophy of epidermis and adnexae together with dermal lymphohistocytic infiltrate. (Courtesy of Dr T. I. Macleod.)

be multiple (Fig. 3.2) and in the scalp cause scarring alopecia (Fig. 3.3). The lips are commonly involved (Fig. 3.2c). Plaque-like lesions may be found on the hard palate and buccal mucosa, sometimes resembling lichen planus. Conjunctival involvement also occurs.

Variants include verrucous LE (Fig. 3.4), especially in the African, chilblain LE (Fig. 3.5) and LE profundus (panniculitis) (Fig. 3.6).

Facial lesions of discoid LE should be distinguished

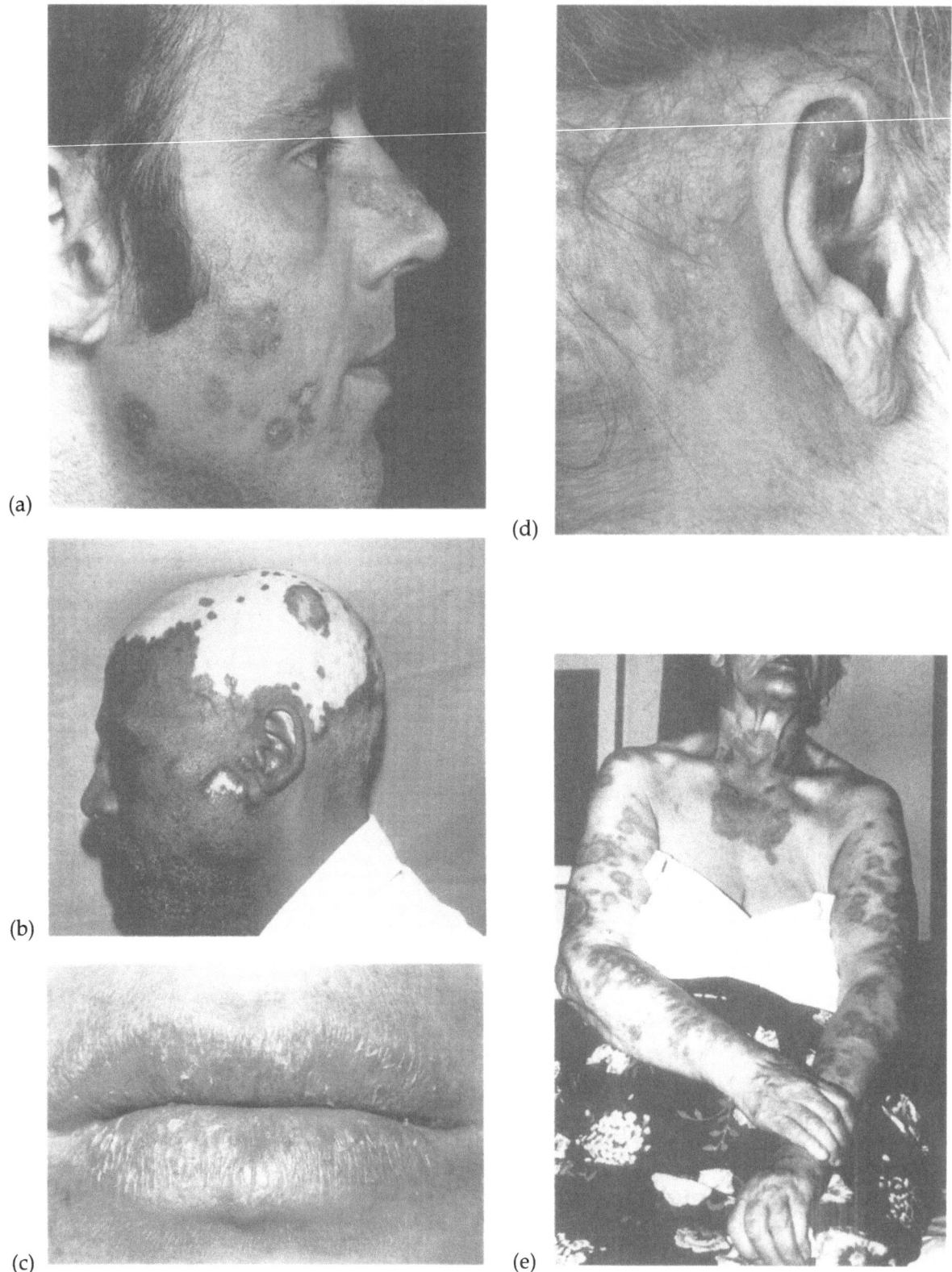

Fig. 3.2 Discoid erythematosus. (a) Typical lesions on the cheek and nose showing atrophic scarring and focal hyperkeratosis. (b) Extensive hypopigmented lesions in negroid skin. (c) Involvement of lips. (d) Involvement of external ear and adjacent scalp. (e) Widespread discoid LE affecting light-exposed areas. ((b) and (e) courtesy of Dr S. O'Langhlin.)

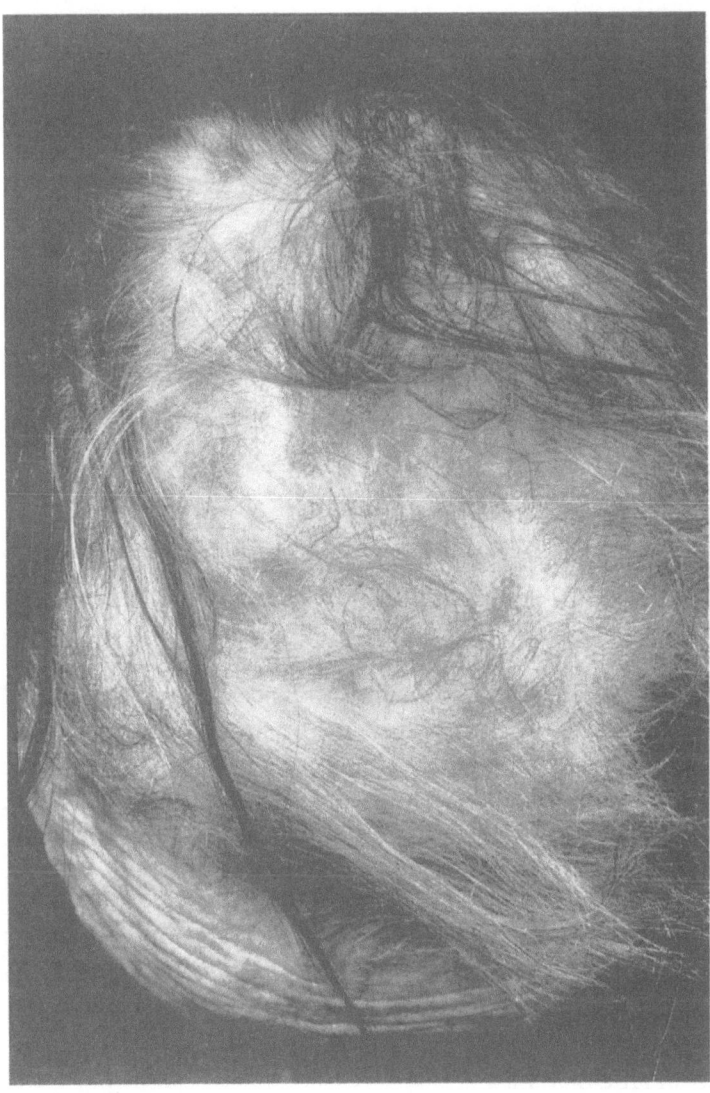

Fig. 3.3 Scarring alopecia in discoid LE; areas of follicular plugging are present.

from confluent areas of rosacea, in which pustules are usually found and from psoriasis in which typical lesions are usually encountered elsewhere. Chilblain LE may be indistinguishable from erosive lichen planus and the two conditions sometimes coexist. Lupus vulgaris presents as solitary or a few asymmetrically distributed plaques on the head and neck. Compression with a glass slide typically reveals the characteristic 'apple jelly' nodules. Other granulomatous conditions which should be excluded are sarcoid, atypical forms of necrobiosis

Fig. 3.4 Verrucous LE; isolated lesions may mimic keratoacanthoma, hypertrophic lichen planus or prurigo nodules. (Courtesy of Dr R. S-H. Tan.)

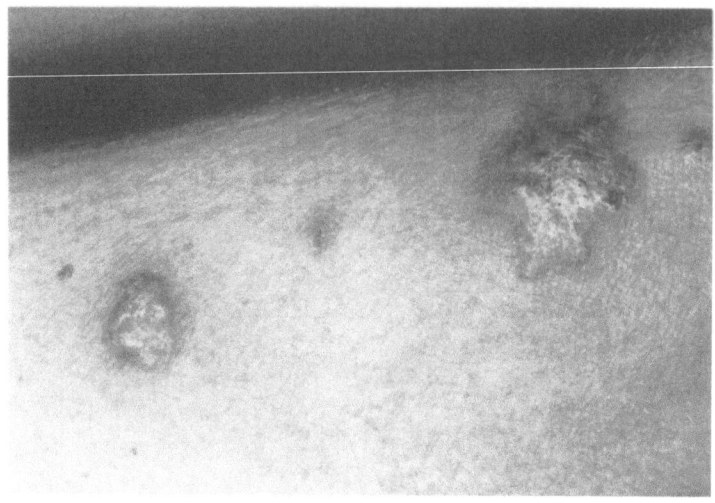

lipoidica and tuberculoid leprosy. Polymorphic light eruption is characteristically transient, each attack lasting only a few days, and tends to spare the face. Superficial basal carcinoma most commonly occurs on the trunk. Although it can form extensive plaques, a raised edge is usually detectable. A skin biopsy is essential if the clinical diagnosis is in doubt.

In discoid LE systemic manifestations are minimal and transient and commoner in the profundus group; they include fatiguability, transient pyrexias and arthralgia; 10% develop classical SLE. Epidermal changes and dermal atrophy are striking histological features. (Fig. 3.1b).

3.5 PAPULAR LE

Violaceous, indurated lesions affect the head, neck and upper trunk, typically following exposure to sunlight (Fig. 3.7). Systemic features are rare. The characteristic histological features are a dermal mononuclear cell infiltrate with minimal changes in the basement membrane and epidermis.

Papular LE can be difficult to distinguish clinically from rosacea. In the latter condition telangiectatic pustules are often associated and a skin biopsy of an established lesion reveals numerous granulomata, often around sebaceous glands. Jessner's lymphocytic in-

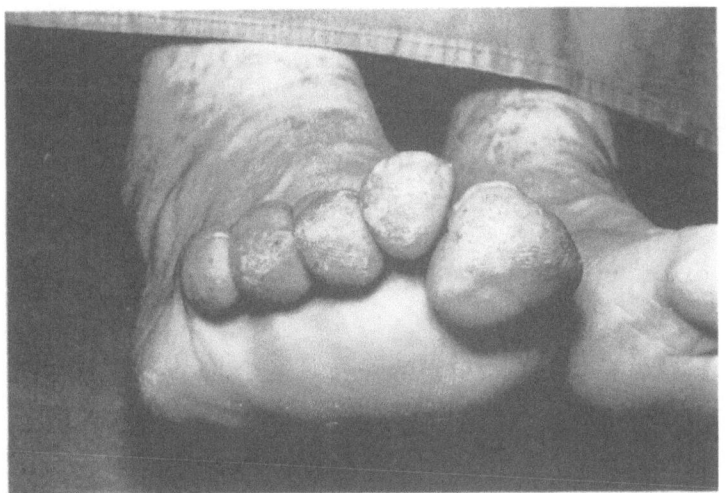

Fig. 3.5 Chilblain LE.
(a) Affecting toes; lesions are usually persistent, unlike simple chilblains. (b) Affecting nose.

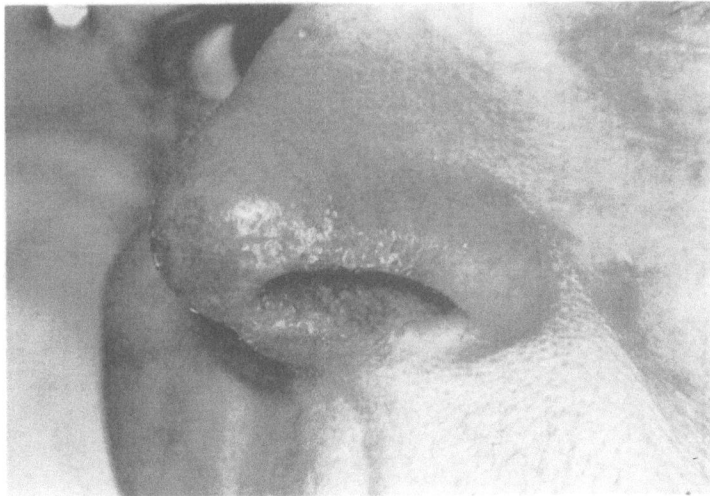

filtrate usually presents as arcuate areas of violaceous erythema and histology typically shows pronounced infiltration of lymphocytes apparently forming follicles in the dermis.

In pemphigus erythematosus (Senear–Usher syndrome) a hyperkeratotic facial eruption, which may mimic seborrhoeic dermatitis, is associated with flaccid bullae or crusts on the trunk. Direct immunofluorescence

Fig. 3.6 Lupus profundus. Predominantly affects cheeks and proximal limbs presenting as tender subcutaneous induration often associated with an overlying discoid lesion. (Courtesy of Dr C. T. C. Kennedy.)

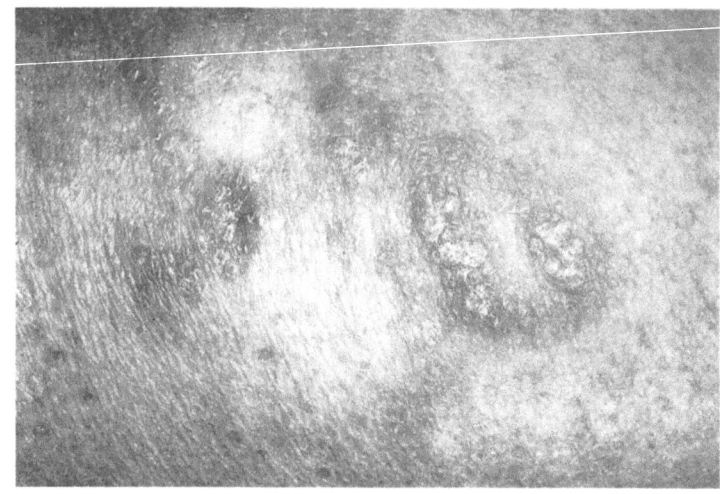

Fig. 3.7 Papular LE: circumscribed erythematous papules with minimal epidermal involvement. Lesions may closely resemble rosacea.

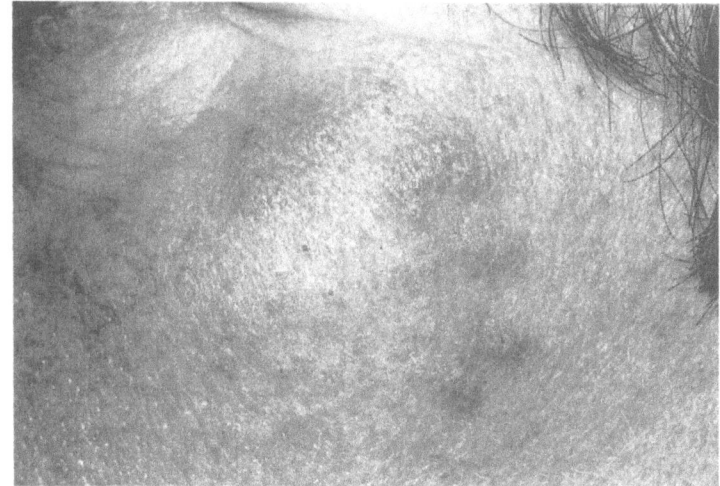

reveals combined features of the lupus band with intercellular immunofluorescence typical of pemphigus. The pathogenesis of the condition is unclear.

3.6 SUBACUTE CUTANEOUS LE

This occurs classically in the caucasian often with a later age of onset. The skin is predominantly involved and lesions often follow ultraviolet exposure. There are widespread annular or papulosquamous (psoriasiform)

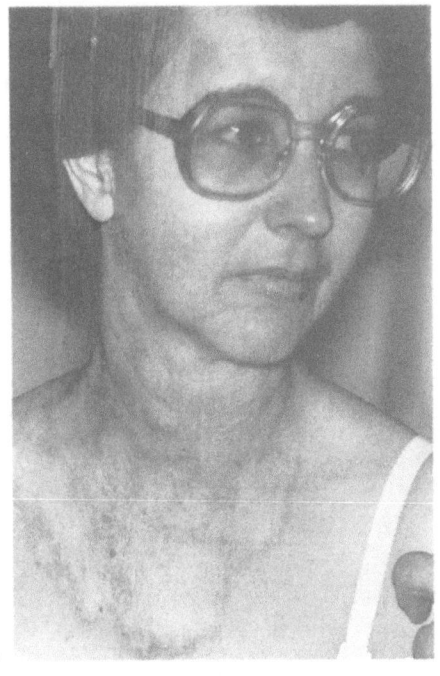

(a)

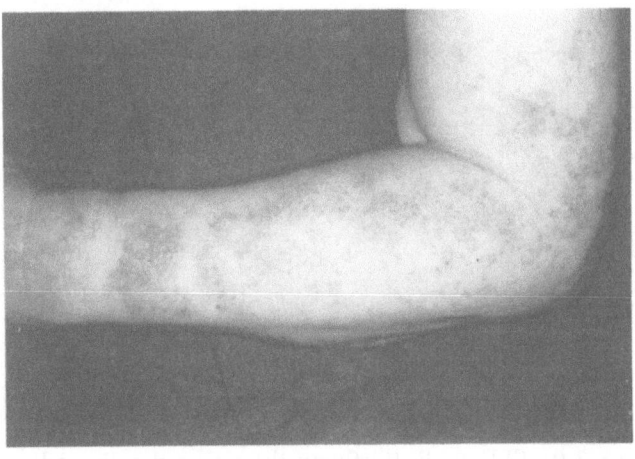

(b)

Fig. 3.8 SCLE. (a) Annular lesions – sometimes these may mimic dermal erythema multiforme (Rowell's syndrome) (courtesy of Dr R. Sontheimer). (b) Papulosquamous lesions may sometimes mimic psoriasis; however lesions are characteristically restricted to light-exposed areas.

erythematous infiltrated lesions that resolve with minimal scarring (Fig. 3.8). The annular infiltrated lesions may mimic the dermal form of erythema multiforme and have been termed Rowell's syndrome. Mild systemic symptoms, such as arthralgia, are common, but major renal and CNS complications are rare.

Histology is characterized by marked liquefaction degeneration, dermal oedema and often florid lymphocytic infiltration of the dermis (Fig. 3.1a). Epidermal changes are rare.

3.7 SYSTEMIC LE

Skin lesions are common but may be transient and episodic – reflecting disease activity. Frequently seen are butterfly erythema (Fig. 3.9a), exanthemata, diffuse alopecia (Fig. 3.9b) and shallow, painless mucosal ulceration. There may be features of discoid LE (10%). Small vessel vasculitis leads to palpable purpura, livedo

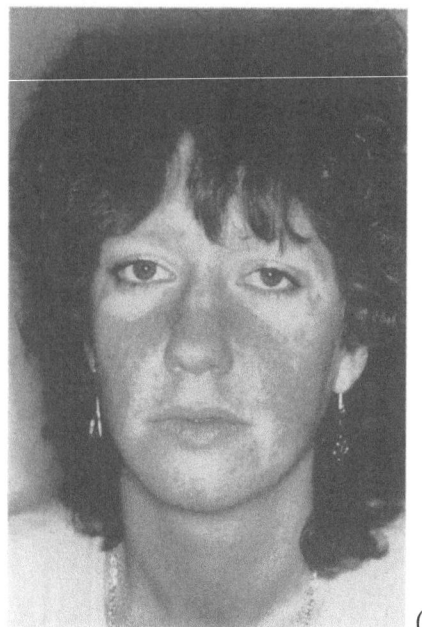

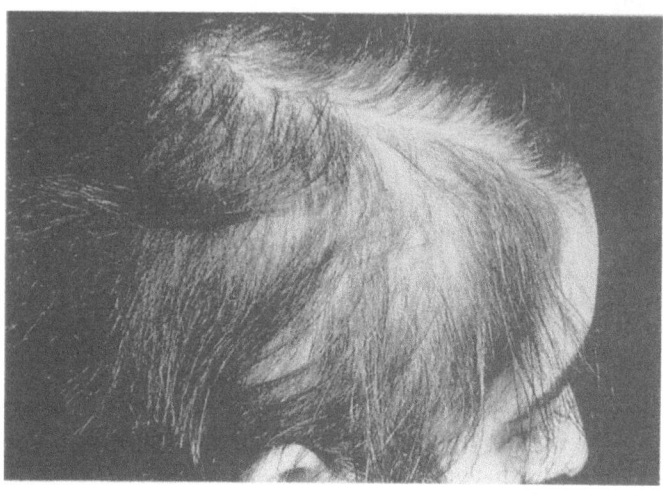

(a)　　　　　　　　　　　　　　(b)

Fig. 3.9　SLE. (a) Butterfly erythema on cheeks and nose. (b) Non-scarring alopecia.

reticularis (see Plate 1), digital lesions (Fig. 3.10) and, less commonly, urticaria-like lesions. Small vessel infarcts in the skin may present as ivory white areas of atrophic blanche, also seen in Degos' syndrome. Rarely, large vessel involvement results in gangrene. Purpura due to thrombocytopenia and bullous lesions are rare.

Table 3.6　Clinical manifestations of SLE

Manifestation	Per cent
Arthritis	90
Skin changes	80
Fever	80
Renal disease	50
Pleurisy	40
Lymphadenopathy	40
Raynaud's	30
Neuropsychiatric disease	30
Alopecia	30
Pericarditis	30
Mouth ulcers	30

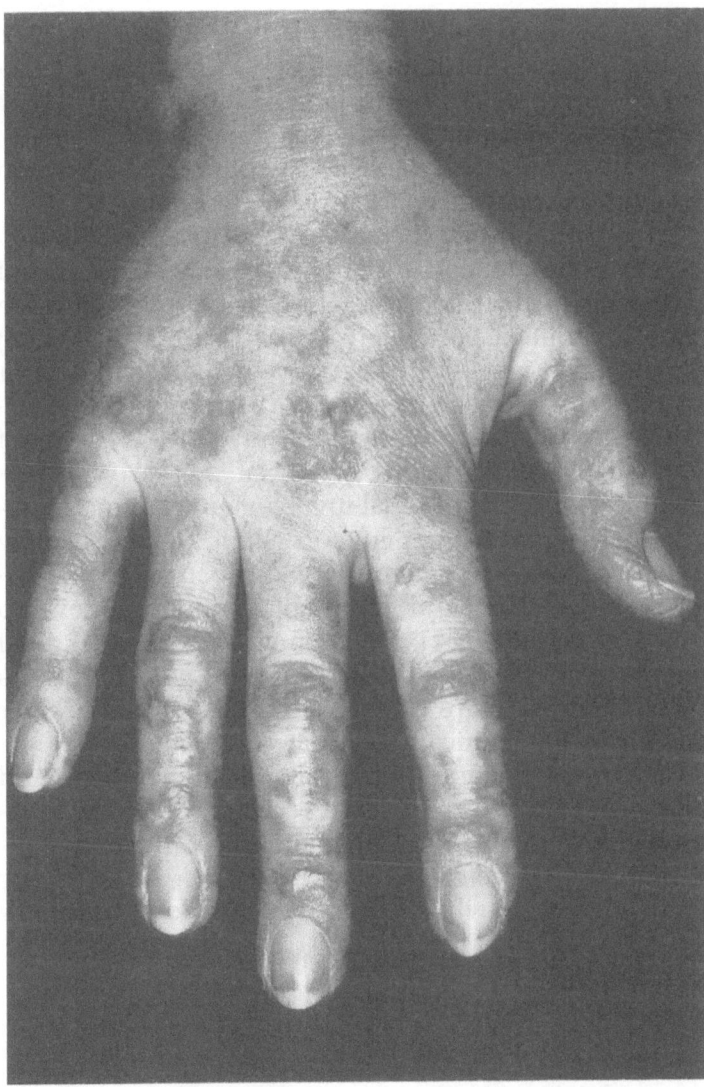

Fig. 3.10 Vasculitic lesion in SLE: digital vasculitis.

Raynaud's may be severe in some individuals, often as-sociated with sausage fingers and occasionally frank sclerodactyly. Nail changes are usually associated with longstanding Raynaud's; there may be violaceous colouring of the nail plate with periungual erythema, longitudinal ridging and crumbling of the nail.

The frequency of systemic features is shown in Table 3.6. At presentation the most common features are musculoskeletal symptoms including painful arthralgia and myalgia, constitutional manifestations, such as fatigue, malaise, fever and loss of weight, and an eruption. A small proportion present in 'lupus crisis' in which extreme weakness and fatigue together with headaches, chest and abdominal pain are accompanied by florid renal or neuropsychiatric involvement.

Polyarthritis occurs commonly and characteristically the symptoms, which are often very severe, are out of proportion to objective signs of synovitis. A few develop joint deformities particularly of the hands (Fig. 3.11) and feet. These result from involvement of periarticular structures and resemble Jaccoud's arthropathy associated with chronic rheumatic fever. Bony erosions of the joints are uncommon.

Clinical evidence of renal involvement is found in approximately half the patients, in whom there is usually mild to moderate proteinuria accompanied by microscopic haematuria and casturia. A minority develop severe proteinuria, hypertension and progressive renal insufficiency. Histological indicators of poor prognosis for renal function are extensive glomerular and tubular scarring with significant vascular involvement.

Headaches, sometimes migrainous, are common and other features of CNS disease occur in more than one-third. CNS involvement is commonly diffuse and includes neuropsychiatric manifestations and organic brain syndromes which can be severe. However, these

Fig. 3.11 Arthritis in SLE. Considerable joint deformities result from periarticular involvement.

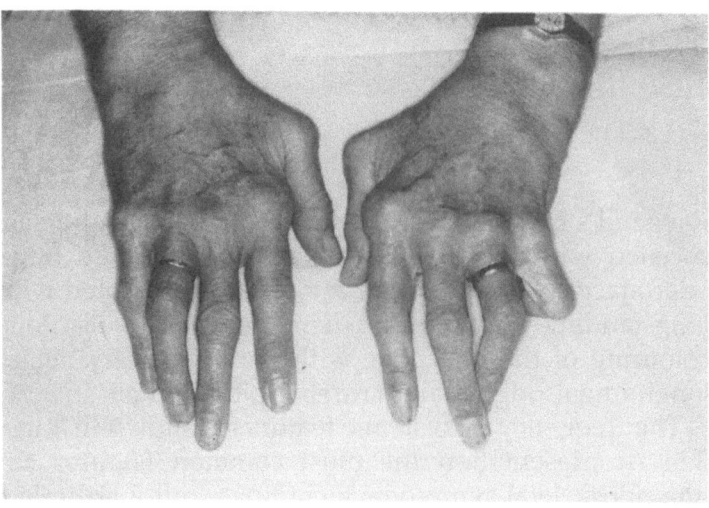

are usually transient leaving minimal residual deficit. Less commonly, serious focal disturbances such as stroke occur leaving persistent disability.

Associations have been noted between lupus and other diseases such as myasthenia gravis and porphyria cutanea tarda. Individuals with inherited deficiency of early complement components, notably C_2 deficiency, are prone to develop lupus. It is of interest that cutaneous features are prominent in such patients together with the frequent presence of antibodies to Ro(SSA) (see section 3.10).

Certain cutaneous manifestations are associated with particular patterns of systemic disease; for example, livedo reticularis with focal CNS involvement such as stroke; Raynaud's and swollen fingers with pulmonary fibrosis and myositis.

3.8 NEONATAL LE

This is rare, with onset within the first few weeks of life. Transient annular erythema, sometimes with periorbital oedema, occurs often following sun exposure (Fig. 3.12 a and b). Systemic features such as thrombocytopenia may occur. Congenital heart block is another characteristic abnormality which has been diagnosed as early as 22 weeks of gestation and often occurs in the absence of skin disease. Resolution of the eruption occurs usually within 6 months, although heart block is a persistent feature which may require a pacemaker. There is a strong association with maternal antibodies to the ribonucleoprotein antigens Ro and La (see section 3.10) and it is believed that passage of maternal antibody across the placenta has a role in the pathogenesis of neonatal lupus. Mothers may have clinical features of SLE or Sjögren's syndrome, but in 50% of cases they are asymptomatic at the time of delivery. However, many develop a connective tissue disease later in life.

3.9 DIAGNOSIS

3.9.1 Differential diagnosis

Differential diagnosis of cutaneous lupus erythematosus is summarized in Table 3.7.

Fig. 3.12 Neonatal LE.
(a) Annular lesion following
sun exposure (courtesy of Dr T.
Provost). (b) Periorbital oedema
(raccoon sign). Note scaling
erythema affecting eyelids and
forehead. (Courtesy of Dr S. K.
Jones.)

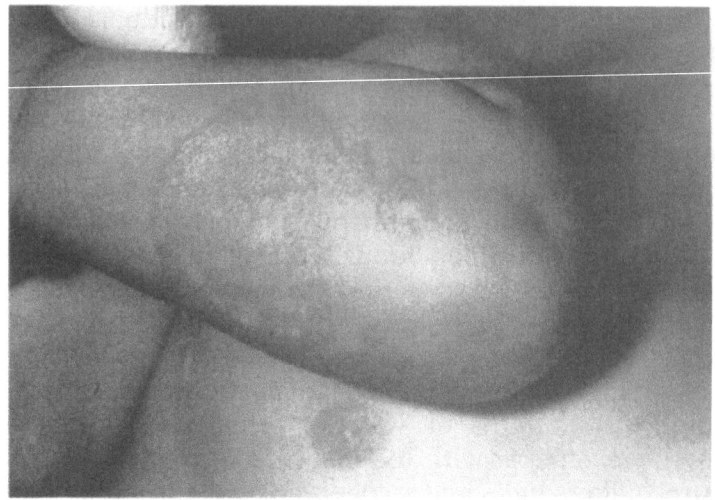

(a)

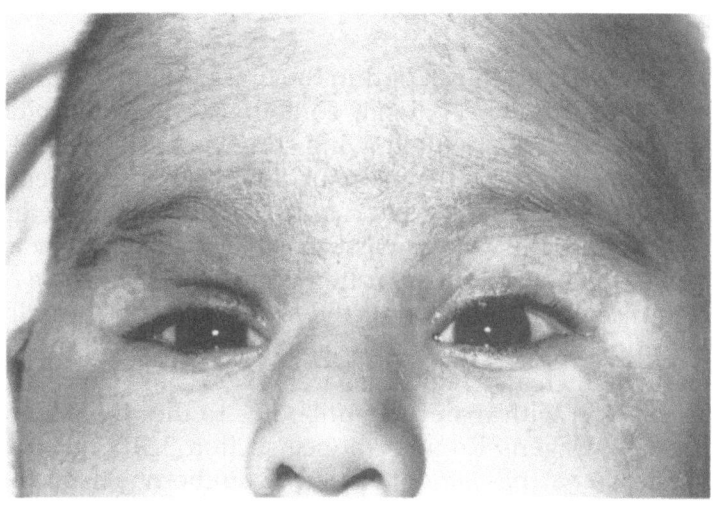

(b)

The diagnosis of SLE depends on recognizing a characteristic pattern of clinical and laboratory abnormalities.
Table 3.8 shows the criteria for SLE revised by the
American Rheumatism Association in 1982. A combination of the features discriminates SLE from other
conditions although the criteria were designed for classification and for use in clinical and therapeutic studies
rather than for bedside diagnosis.

Table 3.7 Differential diagnosis of cutaneous LE

(1) Discoid lesions: psoriasis, superficial basal cell carcinoma, granulomata, for example, TB (lupus vulgaris) and leprosy
(2) Chilblain LE: chilblains and erosive lichen planus
(3) Papular: rosacea, lymphocytic infiltrates, for example, Jessner's
(4) SCLE: erythema multiforme, psoriasis
(5) Photosensitivity: polymorphic light eruption, drug induced photosensitivity, erythrohepatic protoporphyria, xeroderma pigmentosum
(6) SLE butterfly rash: rosacea, drug induced photosensitivity
(7) Alopecia: patchy – alopecia areata, psoriasis, syphilis
diffuse – metabolic (for example, thyroid disease, iron deficiency)

Table 3.8 Revised (1982) ARA criteria for SLE*

(1) Malar rash
(2) Discoid rash
(3) Photosensitivity
(4) Oral ulcers
(5) Non-erosive arthritis
(6) Pleurisy or pericarditis
(7) Renal disorder: (a) persistent proteinuria (>0.5 g/day)
or (b) cellular casts
(8) Neurological disorder: seizures or psychosis
(9) Haematological disorder: (a) haemolytic anaemia
or (b) leukopenia ($<4 \times 10^9$/l) on two occasions
or (c) lymphopenia ($<1.5 \times 10^9$/l) on two occasions
or (d) thrombocytopenia ($<100 \times 10^9$/l)
(10) Immunological disorder: (a) positive LE cells
or (b) antiDNA
or (c) antiSm
or (d) false positive VDRL
(11) ANA

* Four or more criteria required for diagnosis of SLE

Table 3.9   Features characterizing SLE

Female aged 15–35
Typical involvement of skin and mucous membranes
Polyarthritis: painful, non-erosive, often seronegative
Serositis
Immune complex nephritis
Diffuse CNS disease
Lymphopenia, thrombocytopenia
Positive ANA test
Antibodies to certain nuclear antigens, such as DNA, Sm

Fig. 3.13   Lupus band test showing granular deposition of immunoglobulins at dermo-epidermal junction. Note that this must be distinguished from the background staining of the dermal collagen.

Table 3.9 outlines pointers to the diagnosis of SLE in clinical practice.

3.9.2   Investigations helpful for diagnosis and prognosis

These are summarized as follows:

(1) Histology of a skin lesion can be diagnostic.
(2) Skin immunofluorescence; discoid LE is positive in lesional skin, negative in normal skin. SCLE is often negative in both. In SLE the lupus band test is positive in non-involved skin (for example, extensor surface of forearm) in 70% of cases (Fig. 3.13).

3.10 SEROLOGY

This is shown in Table 3.10.

(1) Antinuclear antibody (ANA) (preferably using a cultured cell line as substrate, such as Hep-2 cells) is almost always positive in SLE – frequently in a high titre. Less commonly, low titres are detected in discoid and subacute LE. It should be remembered that a positive test is not specific for LE.

(2) Double stranded DNA antibodies are highly specific for SLE (70%) rare in SCLE and absent in discoid LE. They are infrequent in other connective tissue diseases, such as rheumatoid and systemic sclerosis.

(3) Antibodies to ribonucleoprotein antigens such as Sm, U1RNP, Ro(SSA) and La(SSB) are commonly found in SLE. Antibodies to one or more of the four constituents can be detected by immunodiffusion in approximately 70% of cases.

(4) Anti-Sm is highly specific for SLE and is possibly linked to cutaneous vasculitis. It is found in approximately 30% of Afrocaribbean and Asian SLE patients but only in 8% of caucasian patients.

Table 3.10 Common serological findings in SLE

Findings	*Per cent*
(1) Hypergammaglobulinaemia	80
(2) ANA by immunofluorescence	95
(3) Specific ANA	
(a) to DNA	70
(b) to histones	60
(c) to ribonucleoproteins	70
(incl Sm, U1RNP, Ro(SSA), La(SSB))	
(i) Sm	10–30
(ii) U1RNP	30
(iii) Ro(SSA)	35
(iv) La(SSB)	18
(4) Rheumatoid factor	40
(5) Positive Coombs test	30
(6) Anticardiolipin antibodies	20
(7) False positive VDRL	15
(8) Circulating lupus anticoagulant	15

(5) Antibodies to U1RNP occur in 30% of SLE patients and are a prominent serological feature in patients showing features of MCTD (section 4.2). They occur in 5% of patients with systemic sclerosis but rarely in other clinical conditions.

(6) Antibodies to Ro(SSA) and La(SSA) tend to occur in the same serum. AntiRo is found in 30% of SLE and is the predominant serological abnormality in SCLE (80%) and neonatal lupus. These antibodies also occur in Sjögren's syndrome, occasionally in other connective tissue diseases, but rarely in other clinical conditions or in the normal healthy population (less than 1%).

(7) Anticardiolipin antibodies are found in 20% of SLE patients and high titres of IgG antibodies are associated with livedo reticularis, arterial and venous thrombosis, recurrent abortion and thrombocytopenia. There is a correlation with a false positive VDRL and the lupus anticoagulant.

3.11 TREATMENT

Treatment of cutaneous manifestations is symptomatic. General measures include sunscreens with high protection factor and relevant advice about sun exposure. A variety of sunscreens are readily available. The sun protection factor (SPF) is the ratio of the dose of ultraviolet radiation which produces minimum erythema with sunscreen over that without sunscreen. A standard source of ultraviolet light is used, usually UVB. Protection against long wave ultraviolet light (UVA) is more difficult and thus the SPF is of only partial clinical relevance. Commercially available sunscreens contain mixtures of chemical ultraviolet absorbers, for example, para-aminobenzoic acid, cinnamates and physical barriers such as titanium dioxide or zinc oxide in an oily base. Several preparations are available on prescription for patients with photosensitive disorders. Cosmetic camouflage is useful.

Discoid and papular lesions often require potent topical steroids, perhaps with occlusion. Intralesional steroids may cause scarring.

If topical therapy fails consider antimalarials, for example, hydroxychloroquine and mepacrine (retinal risk minimal but annual ophthalmological assessment is advisable). Other drugs include dapsone (50–100 mg od), oral gold (6 mg od) and thalidomide for chilblain and profundus lesions. Plasmapheresis or pulse therapy with oral or parenteral steroids may be helpful in severe flares but long term systemic steroids and cytotoxic agents are rarely required for cutaneous disease.

Treatment of other manifestations of SLE is also symptomatic with an attempt to limit irreversible pathological damage in vital organs such as the kidney. Drug therapy in mild cases includes non-steroidal anti-inflammatory drugs (NSAIDS). Antimalarials can be very effective for moderately severe disease and their effect extends beyond the treatment of skin disease with suppression of serological parameters in some cases. Alternatively low dose corticosteroids can be effective for features such as severe arthritis, serositis and debilitating constitutional symptoms. Major manifestations such as severe glomerulonephritis and severe CNS and haematological disease initially require high dose corticosteroids combined with an immunosuppressive agent such as oral azathioprine. Treatment with intravenous pulses of cyclophosphamide in a dose of 15 mg/kg body weight can be both effective and well tolerated in refractory cases.

3.12 PROGNOSIS

The prognosis for life in discoid LE is excellent although skin lesions tend to be chronic, resulting in scarring. In SLE the prognosis is determined by the degree of major organ involvement, for example, of kidneys and CNS, and is not adversely affected by the degree of cutaneous involvement.

BIBLIOGRAPHY

Dubois, E. L. (1974) *Lupus Erythematosus: a review of the current status of discoid and systemic lupus erythematosus and their variants* (2nd edn). University of California Press, Los Angeles.
Hughes, G. R. V. (1982) Systemic lupus erythematosus. *Clinics in Rheumatic Diseases.* 8 April:1.
Morrow, J. and Isenberg, D. (1987) *Autoimmune Disease.*

Blackwell, Oxford.

Rothfield, N. F. (1981) Clinical features of systemic lupus erythematosus, in *Textbook of Rheumatology* (eds Kelly, W. N., Morris, E. D. Jr, Ruddy, S. and Sledge, C. B.), Saunders, Philadelphia, **11**, pp. 1106–32.

CHAPTER FOUR

Dermatomyositis and overlap syndromes

4.1 DERMATOMYOSITIS

The term dermatomyositis describes the association between a characteristic eruption and myositis. It is rarer than lupus erythematosus (LE) and systemic sclerosis and the female predominance is less marked. It can occur at any age, predominantly from the fifth decade, but distinct forms occur in children.

4.1.1 Clinical features

Periorbital oedema and violaceous ('heliotrope') erythema affect both upper and lower lids (see Plate 2). Dusky erythema (see Plate 3) occurs on light exposed areas and extensor surfaces which may develop telangiectasia and atrophy (poikiloderma). Hypopigmented lesions occur in negroid skin (Fig. 4.1). The characteristic scaly papules (Gottron's) over knuckles with linear erythematous 'streaks' overlying digits contrast with the pattern in LE (Fig. 4.2). There is striking periungual erythema with dilated and distorted nail fold capillaries with extravasation of blood into a ragged cuticle (Fig. 4.3). These lesions may be precipitated by sun exposure. Scarring alopecia may mimic discoid LE. Calcinosis is a late feature and is more extensive than in systemic sclerosis. Histology of the skin is similar to LE although basement membrane changes are less marked and mucin deposition in the dermis may be a feature (see Plate 4).

Myositis predominantly affects proximal muscles and its severity is not related to the extent of skin disease. Pain and tenderness are not invariable. However, weakness is the cardinal feature usually developing over weeks or sometimes more insidiously. It is apparent using simple tests. These include lifting the head from

Fig. 4.1 Hypopigmented lesion on the knee in a negroid subject. (Courtesy of Dr C. T. C. Kennedy.)

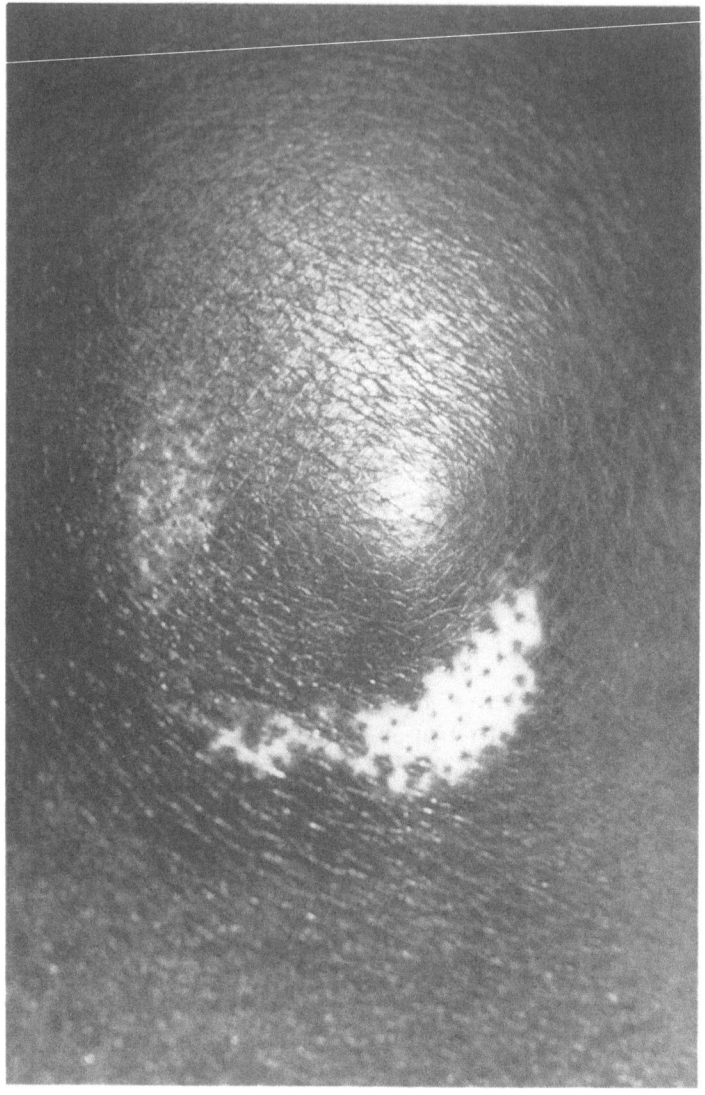

the pillow, raising arms above the head or sitting up and rising from a low chair unaided. Subsequently muscle wasting develops. In severe cases there is difficulty swallowing; respiration may be impaired and may be life-threatening. Constitutional symptoms may be prominent and other systemic features include arthritis and Raynaud's (especially in overlap syndromes) and interstitial lung disease.

Two distinct patterns occur in children, one resembling the adult form, following a chronic course and often

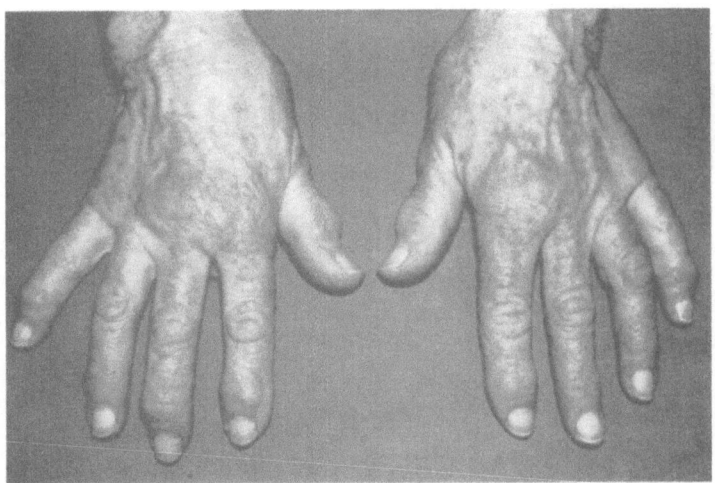

(a)

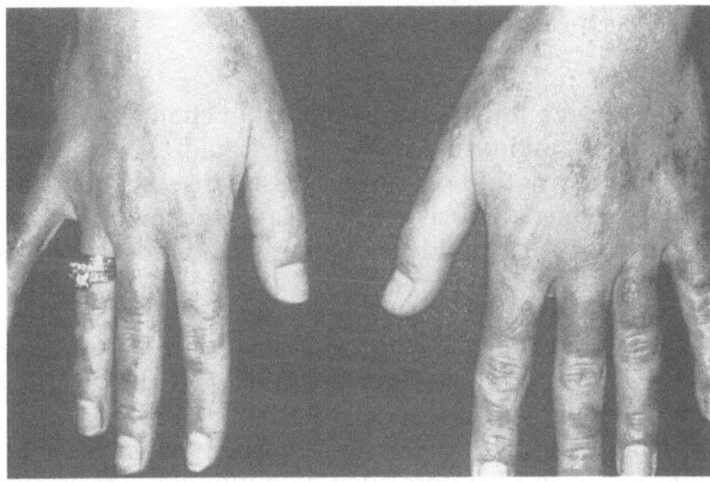

(b)

Fig. 4.2 Contrasting sites of involvement: (a) Dermatomyositis: overlying digits and knuckles. (b) LE: sparing knuckles.

complicated by severe joint contractures and widespread calcinosis (Fig. 4.4). The other is an acute and fulminating disease with vasculitis.

4.1.2 Differential diagnosis

Persistent periorbital oedema should be distinguished from allergic contact dermatitis, systemic LE and Graves' disease. The eyelid changes in angioedema are transient,

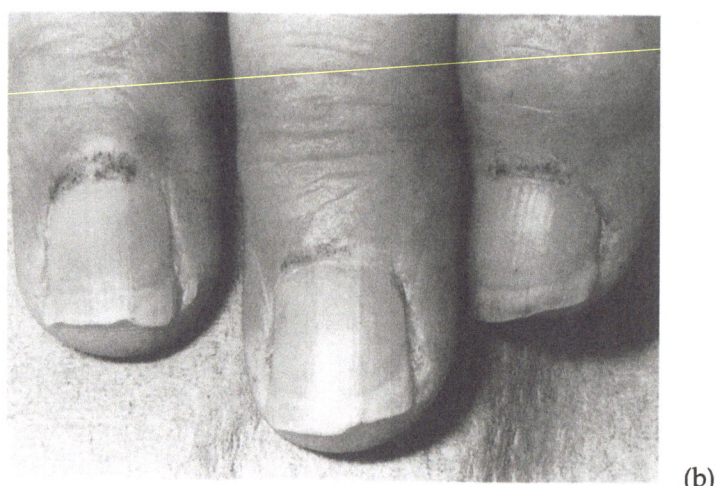 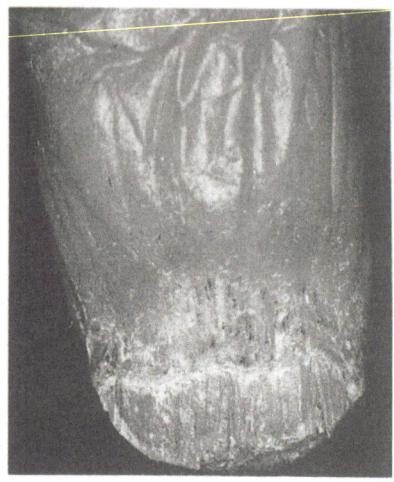

(a)   (b)

Fig. 4.3 (a) The nail fold in dermatomyositis showing ragged cuticle with dilated nail fold capillaries. Small scaly plaques around the nail margins. (b) More severe nail involvement, with obliteration of the nail fold and resorption of the terminal digit.

resolving in a few hours. Similar skin changes occur in trichiniasis. Abnormally dilated nail fold capillaries are also found in other connective tissue diseases, particularly systemic sclerosis and overlap syndromes.

Muscle pain should be distinguished from arthritis and polymyalgia rheumatica (PMR). PMR occurs in the elderly; painful stiff limb girdle muscles are characteristic but muscle power is preserved. Myositis can be infective (for example, toxoplasma) and can be a feature of other connective tissue diseases, notably systemic sclerosis. Absence of neurological signs differentiates dermatomyositis from disorders such as multiple sclerosis and motor neurone disease. Differentiation from primary myopathies can be difficult, although family history and distribution of affected muscles should point to the latter. Myopathy is found in metabolic disorders such as hyperthyroidism and hypothyroidism (in which CPK may be grossly elevated) and primary or iatrogenic Cushing's syndrome.

4.1.3 Pathogenesis

Experimental evidence suggests that cell mediated immunity is important in muscle inflammation. The aetiology is unknown although in children and young

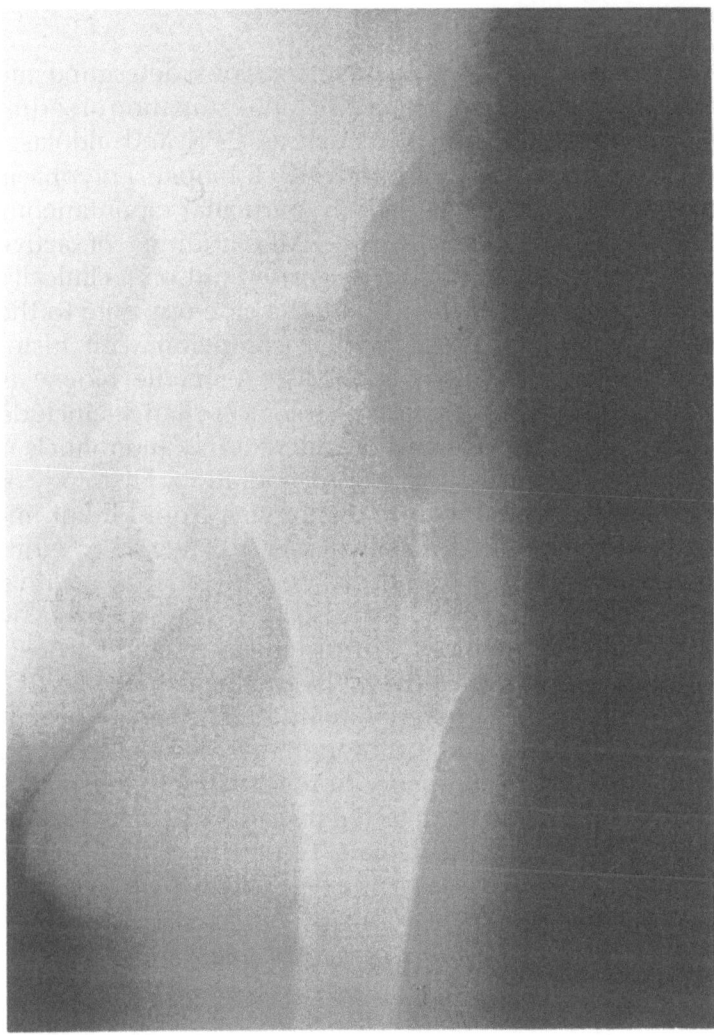

Fig. 4.4 Calcinosis universalis in childhood dermatomyositis. Radiograph showing flecks of calcification in subcutis and muscle. Diffuse calcification typically affects pelvic and shoulder girdles in childhood.

adults there is epidemiological evidence that a Coxsackie virus is implicated. Malignancy is not a feature in this age-group. However, there is a significant association with malignancy in the older patient which is particularly strong in the middle-aged male, when malignancy is found in up to 50%. There is no specific association with particular types of malignancy.

It is current thought that viral or tumour antigens trigger an autoimmune process in a genetically susceptible host. An association, for example, has been reported with HLA DR3.

4.1.4 Investigations

The diagnosis is clinical. Investigations determine the activity of muscle disease and include estimation of serum levels of muscle enzymes such as CPK and aldolase, electromyography (EMG) and muscle biopsy. Polyphasic myopathic potentials and in particular spontaneous fibrillation are characteristic EMG findings of active myositis. A biopsy should be carried out on a clinically abnormal proximal muscle, on the side opposite to the EMG examination. This avoids confusion with histological changes caused by EMG. A needle biopsy is often sufficient and typical histological changes include muscle fibre necrosis and degeneration, a mononuclear cell infiltrate and evidence of regeneration. Histology of the skin can be difficult to distinguish from LE but immunofluorescence is characteristically negative. Nonspecific serological abnormalities include a positive ANA (40%). However, the disease is characterized by antibodies to aminoacyl transferases including Jo-1. Antibodies to Jo-1 (histidyl tRNA synthetase) are specific, occurring in 20%, predominantly in adults without underlying malignancy, although there is an association with interstitial pulmonary fibrosis. Underlying malignancy will usually be detected by careful physical examination including the female genital tract and simple investigations such as chest x-ray. Exhaustive investigation for malignancy is unrewarding.

4.1.5 Treatment and prognosis

Skin lesions may improve with the use of sunscreens and topical steroids; however, systemic treatment is usually required for both skin and systemic disease. Mild cases may respond to antimalarials but most require corticosteroids, initially in high doses (for example, 1 mg prednisolone/kg body weight). Immunosuppressive drugs such as methotrexate are useful for long term therapy as steroid-sparing agents. In the acute stage, frequent respiratory assessment is mandatory, in case assisted respiration is required. In the long term, physiotherapy is essential to avoid contractures. The prognosis is influenced by muscle involvement and underlying malignancy, but not by the extent of skin disease.

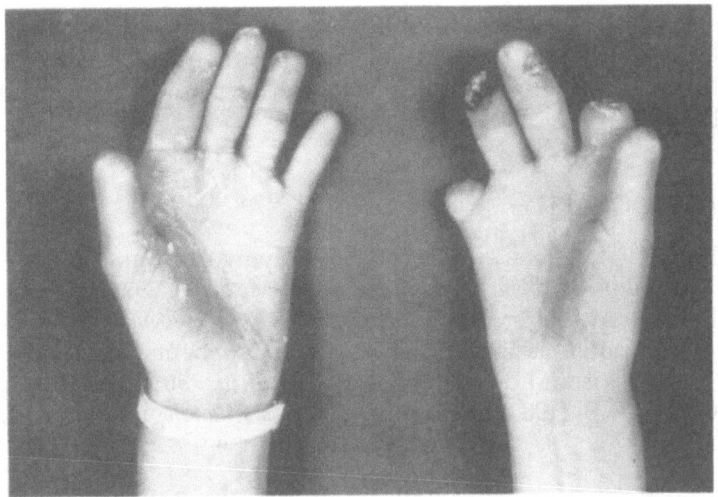

Fig. 4.5 Gangrene of the fingers in a patient with an overlap syndrome.

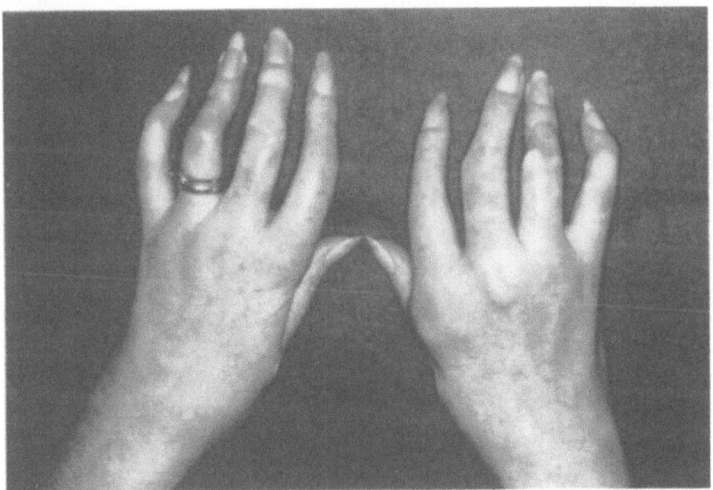

Fig. 4.6 'Sausage' digits in a patient with an overlap syndrome.

4.2 OVERLAP SYNDROMES

Many patients exhibit manifestations of more than one connective tissue disease. Common features are severe Raynaud's phenomenon, sometimes leading to digital gangrene (Fig. 4.5), swollen (sausage) digits (Fig. 4.6) and arthritis. Inflammatory features occur early including myositis and serositis with the subsequent development of sclerodactyly, pulmonary fibrosis and oesophageal involvement in some patients. Significant renal disease is rare. A proportion of these patients have antibodies to U1RNP often as the predominant antibody. This combination of clinical and serological features has been defined as Mixed Connective Tissue Disease.

BIBLIOGRAPHY

Bohan, A., Peter, J. B. (1982) Polymyositis and dermatomyositis. *New England Journal of Medicine*, **292**, 344–483.

Bohan, A., Peter, J. B., Bowman, R. L. *et al.* (1977) A computer assisted analysis of 153 patients with polymyositis and dermatomyositis. *Medicine*, **561**, 255–67.

Callen, J. P. (1983) Dermatomyositis. *Dermatology Clinics* I, **4**, 461–73.

CHAPTER FIVE

Vasculitis

The term vasculitis encompasses a spectrum of disorders in which inflammatory changes occur within the blood vessel wall resulting in vascular obliteration, infarction and haemorrhage. The clinical presentation reflects the size and site of vessel involvement. Until we have a clearer idea of the underlying mechanisms vasculitis is best classified on clinicopathological criteria since these have prognostic implications. On this basis there are three broad groups (Table 5.1); necrotizing vasculitis (section 5.1), small vessel vasculitis (section 5.2) and large vessel arteritis (section 5.3).

In most cases the aetiology is unknown. It is thought, however, that immunopathogenic mechanisms have an important role. The prevailing theory is that polyarteritis nodosa (PAN) is caused by deposition of immune complexes in blood vessel walls. In a proportion there is evidence that immune complexes containing hepatitis B surface antigen (HBAg) are involved. The relative proportion of such cases varies in different parts of the world and is related to the prevalance of HBAg carrier status in the population. Thus such cases constitute up to 80% of PAN seen in some parts of the United States,

Table 5.1 Classification of systemic vasculitis

1. Necrotizing vasculitis
    (a) Polyarteritis nodosa (PAN) group, including classical PAN, Churg-Strauss vasculitis, Wegener's granulomatosis, cutaneous PAN
    (b) Vasculitis associated with connective tissue diseases, including rheumatoid arthritis, systemic lupus erythematosus (SLE), polymyositis (especially children)
2. Small vessel vasculitis (leukocytoclastic vasculitis)
3. Large vessel vasculitis
    (a) Giant cell arteritis
    (b) Takayasu's arteritis

France, Hungary and South America, but to less than 10% of cases in the United Kingdom. Cases of PAN have been associated with acute serous otitis media, polychondritis, hairy cell leukaemia and intravenous methamphetamine abuse. An immune complex mechanism has also been implicated in vasculitis associated with other connective tissue diseases. Complexes comprising of aggregated IgG and IgM rheumatoid factors, for example, have been implicated in vasculitis occurring in rheumatoid arthritis. A variety of aetiological factors have been implicated in leukocytoclastic vasculitis including drug hypersensitivity (for example, sulphonamides, penicillin, thiazides, phenylbutazone), food allergy, infection (such as streptococci) and malignancy. Cell mediated immune reactivity may be involved in disorders such as Wegener's granulomatosis, characterized by extravascular granulation tissue, but there has been recent interest in the presence of antineutrophil antibodies in this disorder, particularly in patients with renal disease, which may provide clues to both pathogenesis and aetiology.

5.1 NECROTIZING VASCULITIS

This is a unifying feature involving medium sized and small arteries (Fig. 5.1). The category includes distinctive but rare entities such as polyarteritis nodosa, Churg–Strauss syndrome, Wegener's syndrome and vasculitis

Fig. 5.1 Histology of typical necrotizing vasculitis, showing fibrinoid necrosis of medium sized artery.

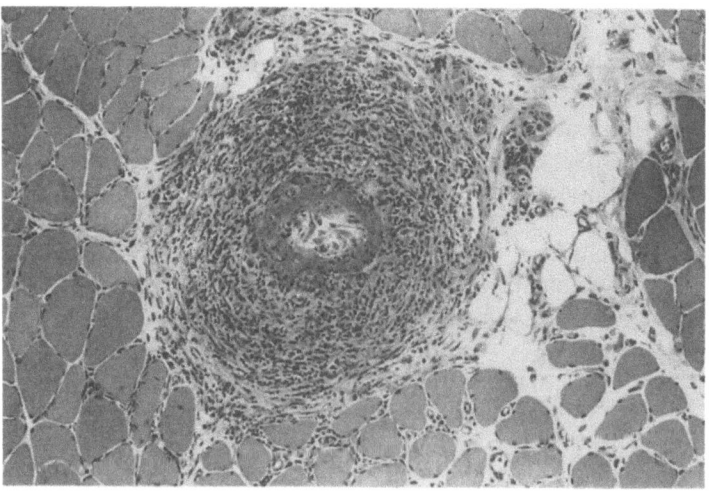

secondary to connective tissue disease such as rheumatoid arthritis. However, there is often overlap.

5.1.1 Polyarteritis nodosa (PAN)

In PAN the process is typically restricted to medium sized and small arteries often with aneurysmal dilatation. The sex incidence is roughly equal and the middle-aged and elderly are affected. Vessel involvement may be widespread leading to a fulminating multisystem disease or may be confined to a single organ such as the skin.

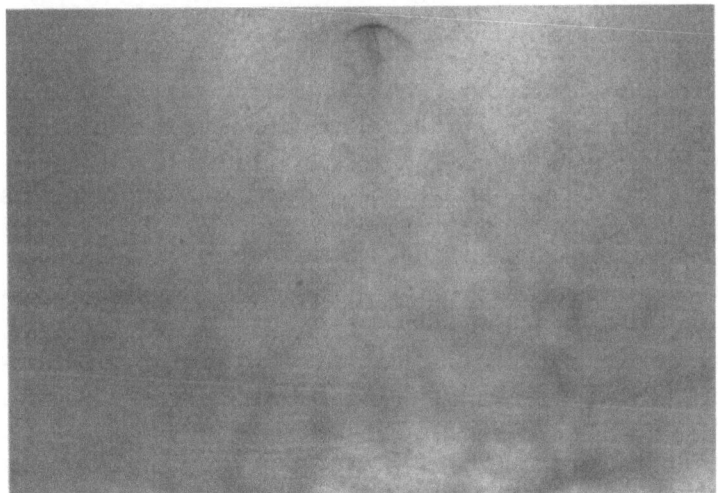

Fig. 5.2 Extensive livedo reticularis in cutaneous polyarteritis.

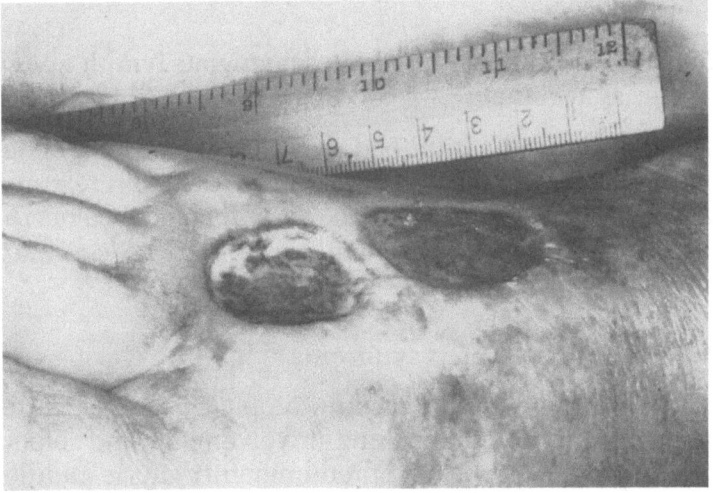

Fig. 5.3 Punched out necrotic ulcer characteristic of arteritis.

Fig. 5.4 Gangrene and haemorrhagic bullae due to polyarteritis nodosa.

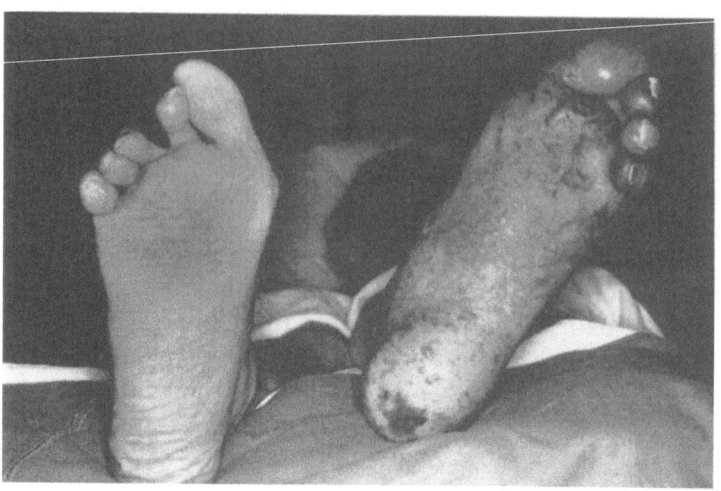

Subcutaneous nodules along the course of arteries, classically described by Kassmaul and Maier, are rarely seen now. More commonly seen are livedo reticularis (Fig. 5.2), punched out necrotic ulcers (Fig. 5.3) and gangrene (Fig. 5.4). Non-specific constitutional symptoms such as weight loss, malaise and pyrexia indicate systemic disease as well as more specific features such as mononeuritis multiplex and renovascular hypertension. Systemic involvement can be confirmed by organ biopsy and/or mesenteric and renal angiography. A primarily cutaneous form occurs in the elderly and in contrast to the systemic form carries a good prognosis. A variant is seen with leg ulceration in the summer months.

5.1.2 Kawasaki disease (mucocutaneous lymph node syndrome)

A virus induced, childhood disorder in which an acute febrile illness with characteristic mucocutaneous features and lymphadenopathy may be accompanied by a necrotizing vasculitis predominantly affecting the coronary arteries.

5.1.3 Churg–Strauss syndrome

Typically there is a preceding atopic history (such as asthma), predominant lung involvement and blood eosinophilia. It is rare and predominantly affects middle-aged males. Skin manifestations include those of PAN together with palpable purpura, reflecting a wider spectrum of vessel involvement. It is the prominence of respiratory tract involvement which distinguishes this condition from classical PAN. Chest x-ray abnormalities such as patchy, shifting infiltrates or bilateral nodular densities are seen in over 50%. Renal involvement is less prominent than in classical PAN but significant cardiac involvement occurs in approximately one-third, eventually leading to cardiac failure.

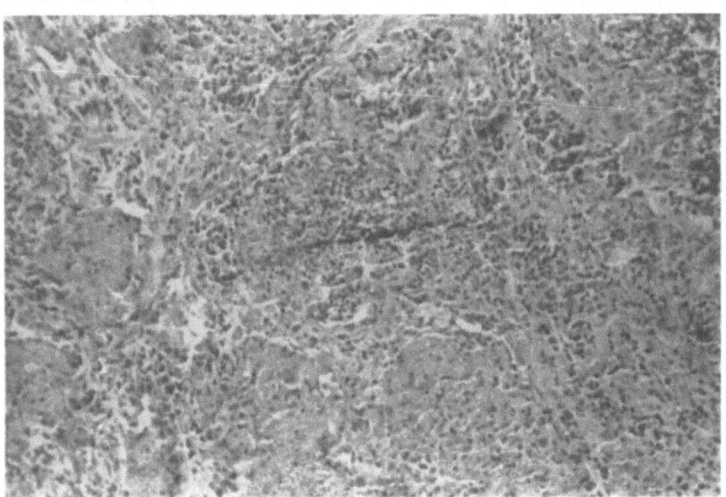

Fig. 5.5 (a) and (b) Pathological features of Wegener's syndrome. Note dense cellular infiltrate affecting small and medium blood vessels. Granulomata are not a characteristic feature.

(a)

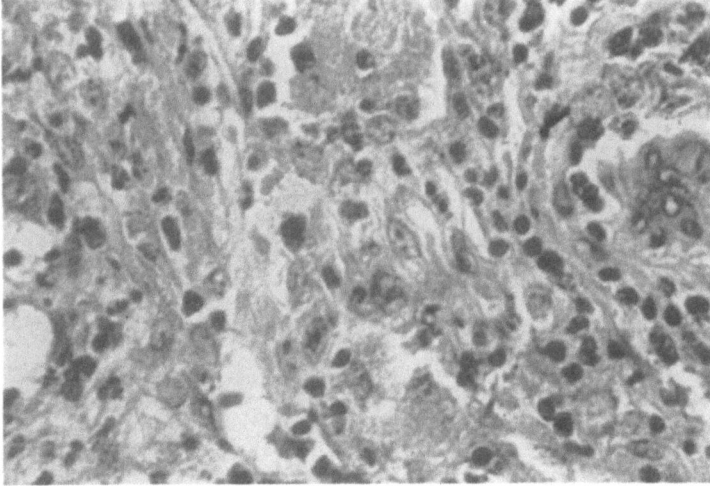

(b)

5.1.4 Wegener's syndrome

The typical pathological feature is a dense mononuclear infiltrate associated with involvement of medium and small vessels (Fig. 5.5). The respiratory tract is invariably involved. The clinical picture results from progressive and destructive inflammation producing, for example, a saddle-nose deformity (Fig. 5.6) and a widespread vasculitis particularly involving the kidneys. As in Churg–Strauss syndrome, the cutaneous manifestations reflect the wide spectrum of vessels involved. Antibodies to a cytoplasmic antigen associated with neutrophil alkaline phosphatase and detected by immunofluorescence are often present and aid diagnosis.

5.1.5 Prognosis and treatment of necrotizing vasculitis

Systemic involvement carries a poor prognosis if untreated but many cases respond to cyclophosphamide.

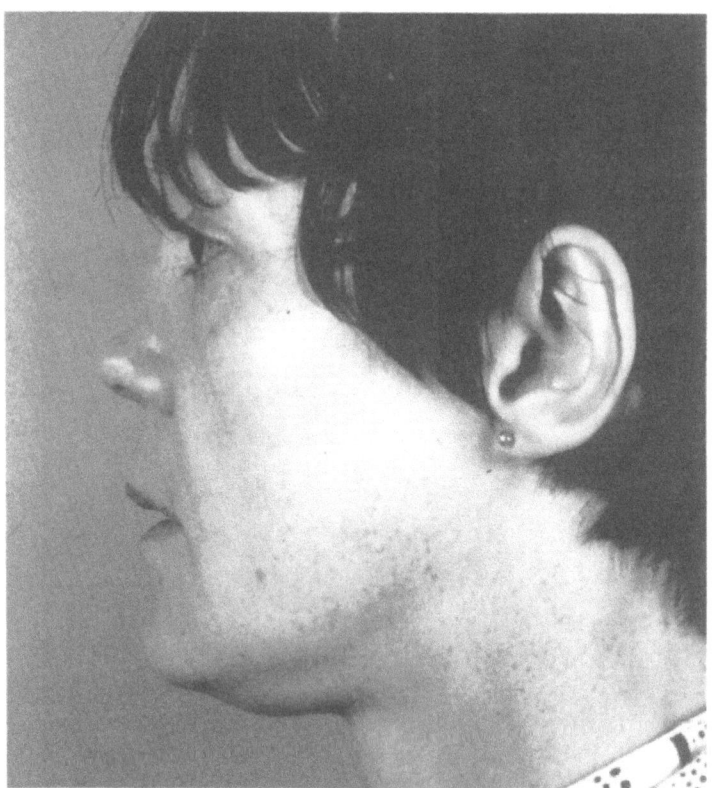

Fig. 5.6 Saddle-nose deformity in Wegener's syndrome. (Courtesy of Prof. P. A. Dieppe.)

Lone skin disease may resolve spontaneously or respond to symptomatic treatment, including bed rest. Some localized cutaneous forms respond well to stanozolol.

5.2 SMALL VESSEL VASCULITIS

This primarily involves the skin and is characterized histologically by involvement of postcapillary venules and capillaries with leucocytoclasis (Fig. 5.7). Painful, palpable purpura occurs especially on dependent parts. Sometimes lesions coalesce, become bullous and ulcerate or they may be urticarial (Fig. 5.8). The aetiology is often

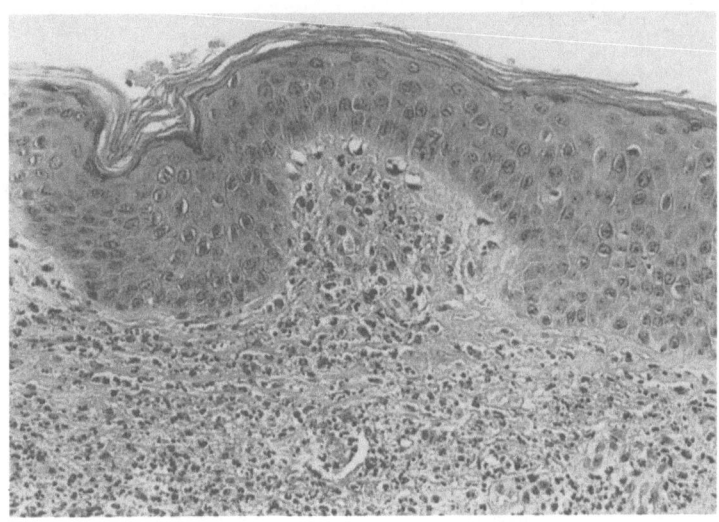

Fig. 5.7 Leucocytoclastic vasculitis showing disrupted venule surrounded by fragmented polymorphs ('nuclear dust'). (Courtesy of Dr T. I. Macleod.)

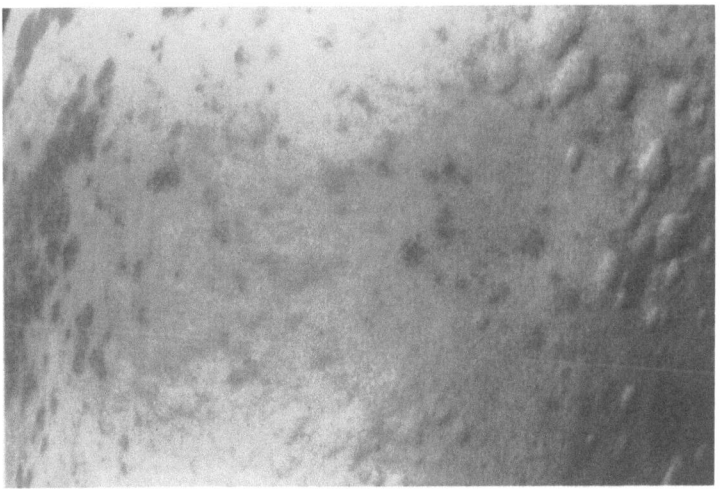

Fig. 5.8 Palpable purpura with urticarial lesions resulting from small vessel vasculitis. (Courtesy of Dr E. Pascual.)

unknown but may follow viral or bacterial infections especially haemolytic streptococci, drugs, such as thiazides and sulphonamides, or malignancy. This group includes two defined syndromes.

Figs. 5.9 and 5.10
Characteristic distribution of Henoch-Schönlein purpura on buttocks and posterior thighs. (Fig. 5.9 Courtesy of Dr Allan St J. Dixon.)

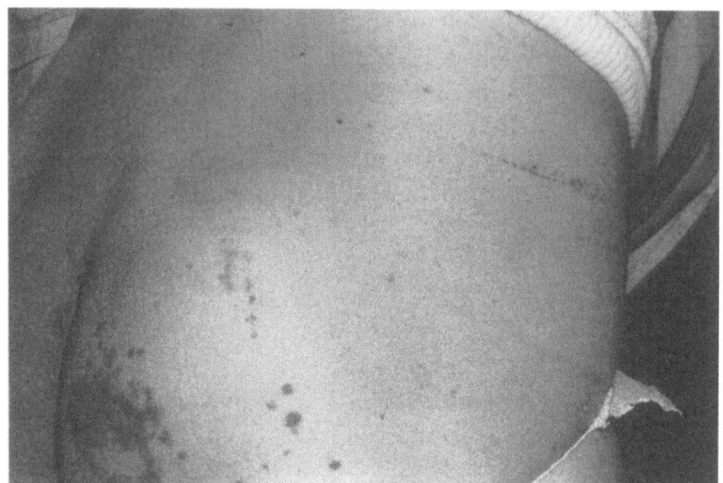

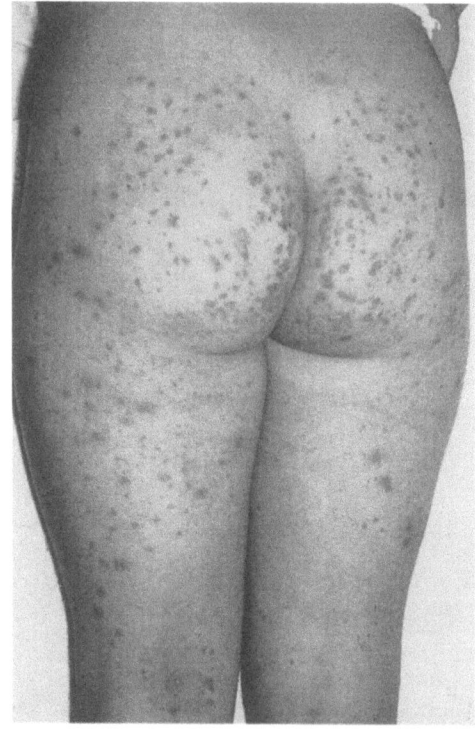

5.2.1 Henoch–Schönlein purpura

This primarily affects children and skin lesions occur chiefly on buttocks and legs (Figs 5.9, 5.10). It may be associated with intussusception, arthralgia and arthritis. Renal involvement may become apparent several weeks after the presentation with skin lesions and occasionally results in renal failure. Henoch–Schönlein purpura is distinguished pathologically by deposition of IgA in affected blood vessels in skin and mesangium.

5.2.2 Essential mixed cryoglobulinaemia

This occurs in middle-aged women, affects the lower legs, and is precipitated by cold. It is associated with aggressive renal disease and characterized by a cryoglobulin consisting of a mixture of IgG and IgM (monoclonal) (Fig. 5.11).

5.2.3 Treatment

Treat the cause if possible. Often no specific treatment is required. Severe Henoch–Schönlein purpura requires

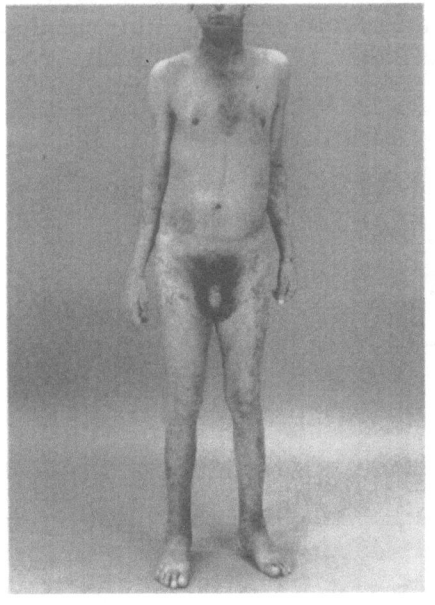
(a)

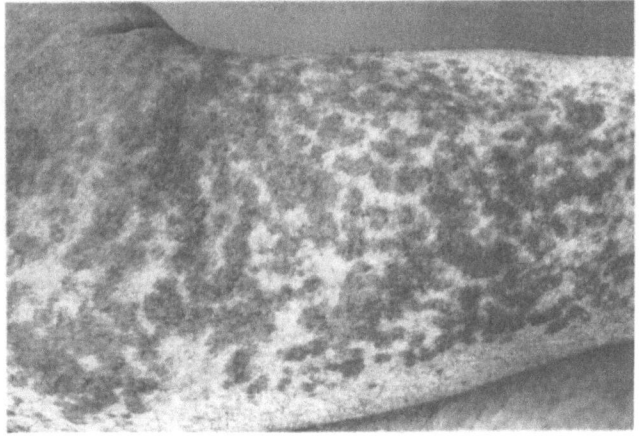
(b)

Fig. 5.11 Widespread cutaneous vasculitis due to essential mixed cryoglobulinaemia. (a) Showing distribution. (b) Morphology of lesions.

systemic steroids or dapsone. Mixed essential cryoglobulinaemia responds poorly to treatment and generally
requires immunosuppression and/or plasmapheresis.

5.3   LARGE VESSEL ARTERITIS

Any large artery may be involved. Histologically there
is a panarteritis with disruption of the internal elastic
lamina, a mononuclear infiltrate and giant cells. Skin
manifestations are not a prominent feature and reflect
ischaemia.

5.3.1   Takayasu's disease

Affects young women, involving the aorta and its major
branches. Raynaud's and trophic changes in the limbs
may occur. Systemic steroids may help.

5.3.2   Giant cell arteritis

This predominantly affects the elderly; there is an equal
sex incidence. It particularly involves branches of the
carotid artery, and temporal artery biopsy can confirm
the diagnosis. Clinical features include unilateral scalp
pain and tenderness, a tortuous nodular non-pulsatile
artery and occasionally scalp infarction (Fig. 5.12). Poly-

Fig. 5.12   Giant cell arteritis
affecting temporal artery.

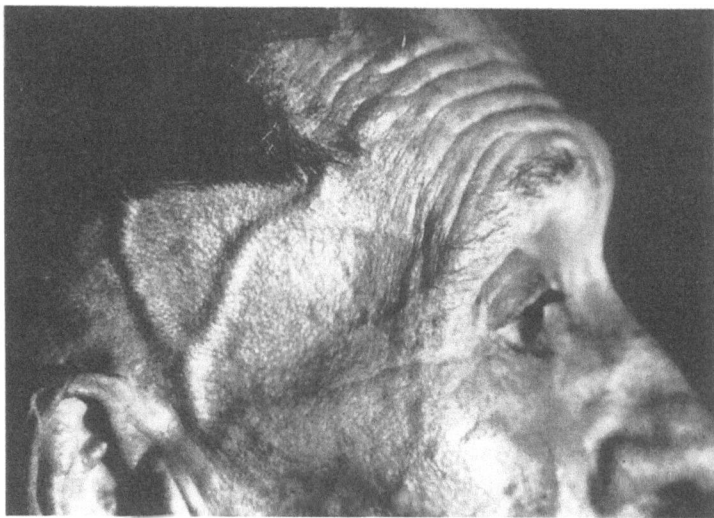

myalgia rheumatica is frequently a presenting feature. Occasionally there is small joint synovitis. Prompt treatment with oral steroids is important to avoid the major complication of blindness.

BIBLIOGRAPHY

Alarcon–Segovia, D. (1980) The necrotizing vasculitides. *Clinics in Rheumatic Diseases*. **August 6**(2).

Fauci, A. S., Haynes, B. F. and Katz, P. (1978) The spectrum of vasculitis. *Annals of Internal Medicine* **89**:660–76.

Fauci, A. S., Haynes, B. F., Katz, P. and Wolff, S. M. (1983) Wegener's granulomatosis: prospective clinical and therapeutic experience with 85 patients for 21 years. *Annals of Internal Medicine*, **98**, 76–85.

CHAPTER SIX

The spondyloarthropathies (psoriatic, enteropathic and other seronegative arthropathies)

6.1 DEFINITION

A number of disorders are broadly grouped as spondyloarthropathies because of common clinical features: a tendency to asymmetrical involvement of large peripheral joints; axial skeleton involvement and enthesopathy (inflammation at the site of bony insertion of ligaments and tendons); systemic features such as uveitis and aortic valve disease; negative rheumatoid factor; strong genetic associations notably with HLA B27; sacroiliitis.

It is probable that the seronegative spondyloarthropathies share a common pathogenesis and that a microbial trigger acts across the mucosa of the bowel or lower urinary tract in a genetically susceptible host.

Ankylosing spondylitis represents the prototype of the seronegative spondyloarthritic syndromes. It shows the closest association with HLA B27 which is present in over 95%. Indeed the prevalence of ankylosing spondylitis in the population around the world relates to the incidence of B27 in the particular ethnic group. Thus in caucasians (HLA B27 in 8%) the prevalence of ankylosing spondylitis is approximately 1%, but the disease is rare in black Africans and Japanese. It occurs in young adults usually in the third decade and although it is most obvious in men, it tends to be underdiagnosed in women and the sex incidence is approximately 2M:1F. The typical presentation is with insidious onset of back pain and stiffness in a young adult. The sacroiliac joint is usually involved first with progression to the lumbar spine ascending to involve each section of the spine in turn. Progressive limitation of spinal movement can occur resulting in disabling flexion deformities of the thoracic and cervical spine in severe and neglected cases. Peripheral joints may be involved, especially the hips and shoulders and insertional tendinitis is a common feature causing, for example, a painful thickened Achilles tendon. Cutaneous manifestations per se are not a feature but systemic features occur and include constitutional symptom of fatigue in most and weight loss and low grade fever in some, anterior uveitis in approximately 25% and, rarely, aortic defects due to subaortic scarring and chronic infiltrative and fibrotic changes in the upper lobes of the lungs.

6.2 PSORIATIC ARTHRITIS

Approximately 7% of patients with psoriasis develop arthritis, representing a significant increase over the general population. Skin involvement precedes arthritis in 75%, but in 20% the reverse holds true. The course

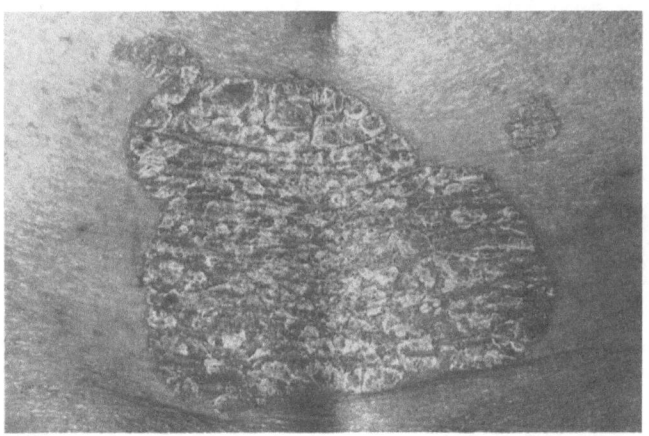

(a)

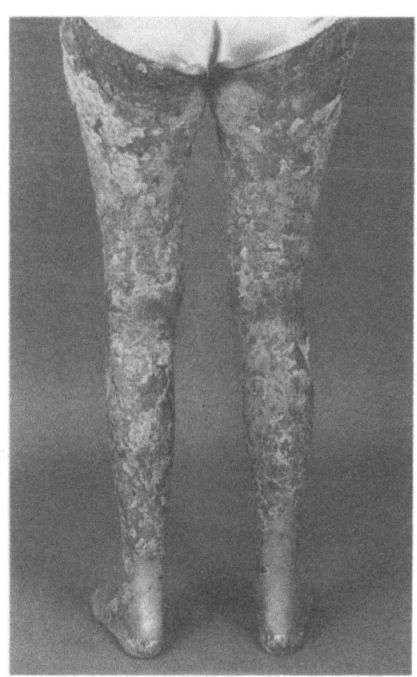

(b)

Fig. 6.1 Psoriatic plaque. (a) Well-demarcated plaque with silvery scales. (b) Extensive plaque psoriasis.

of skin and joint lesions is often independent. Typical plaque psoriasis affects extensor surfaces (Fig. 6.1), but the expression of skin disease is variable. Involvement may be restricted to the scalp, umbilicus, genitalia or gluteal regions. At the other extreme is erythroderma. Pustular psoriasis may be limited to the palms and soles (Fig. 6.2a). Generalized pustular psoriasis (Fig. 6.2b) is rare but severe, and may relate to withdrawal of systemic

Fig. 6.2 Pustular psoriasis. (a) Localized to soles. Note associated hyperpigmented lesions and scale, which may be absent. (b) Generalized. Sheets of small pustules on an erythematous base.

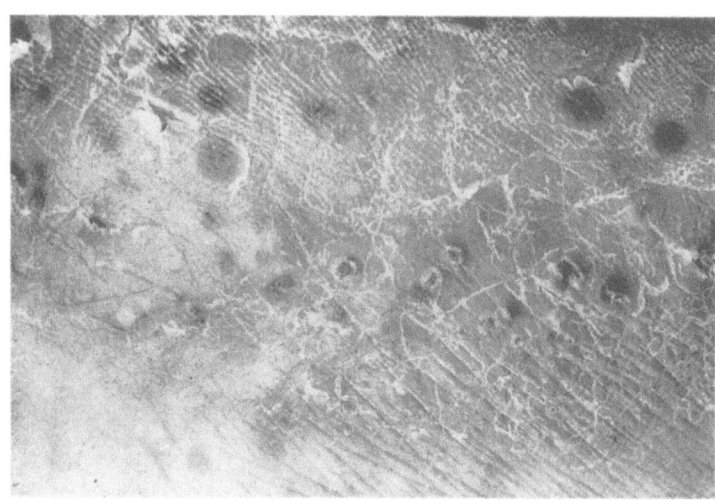

(a)

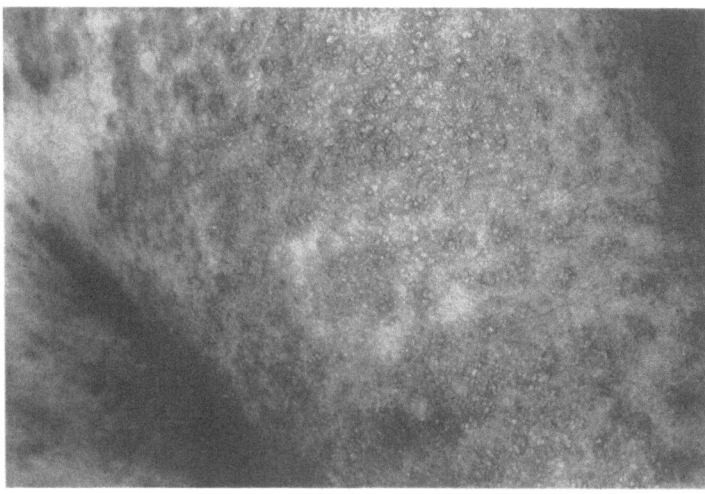

(b)

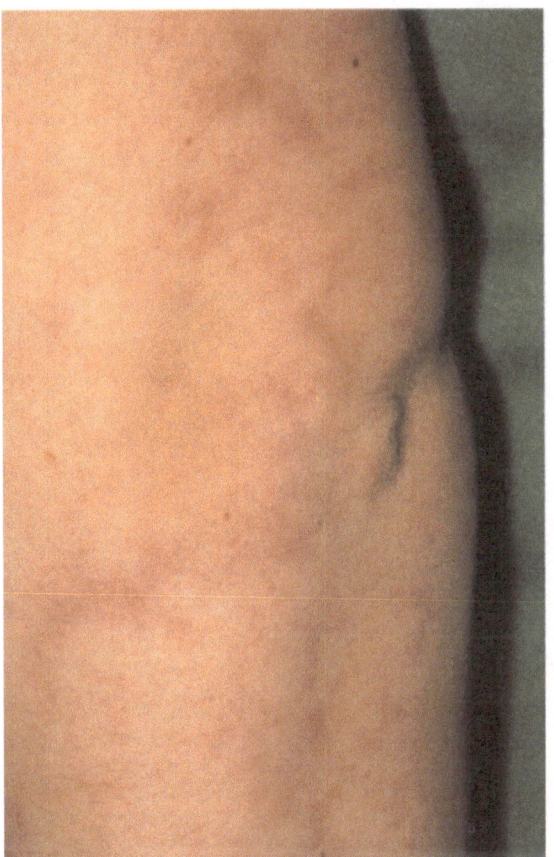

Plate 1 Livedo reticularis lesion in SLE affecting the arm.

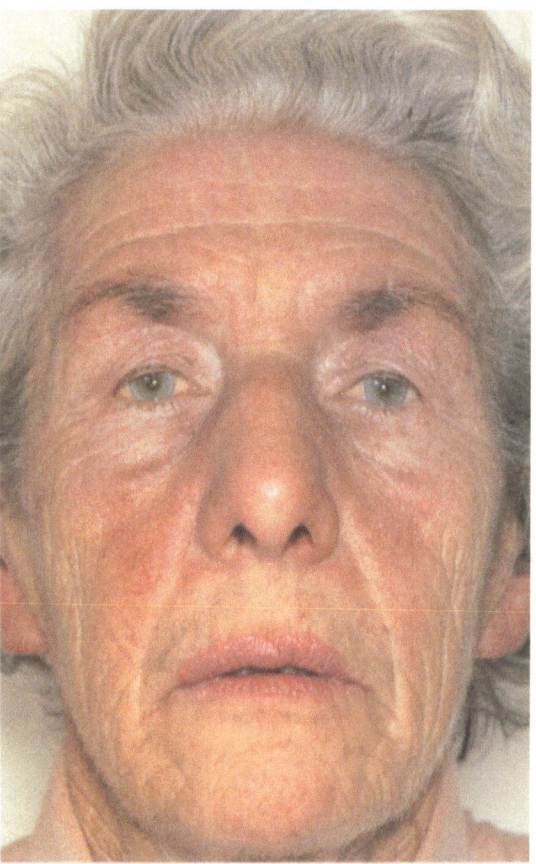

Plate 2 Facial eruption in dermatomyositis showing heliotrope-coloured erythema and oedema of eyelids and photosensitive distribution.

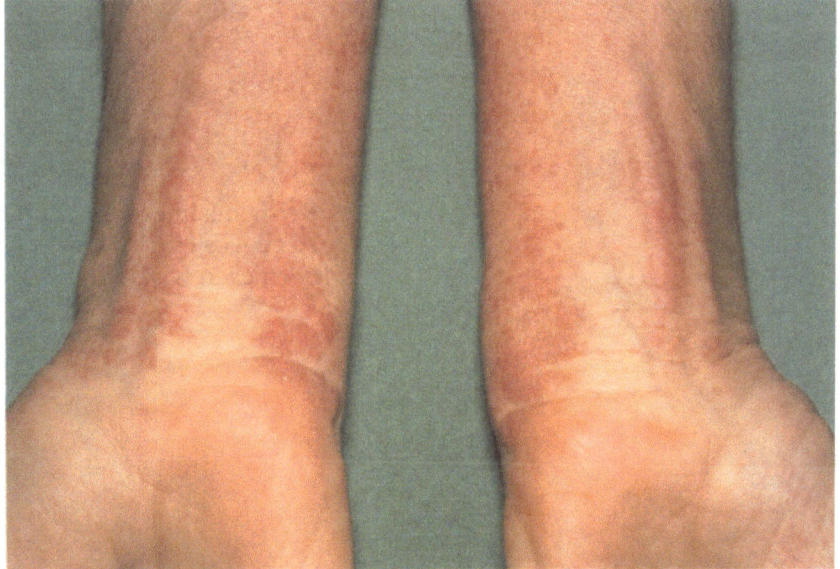

Plate 3 Violaceous erythema on the flexor forearms. Lesions occur more typically on extensor surfaces.

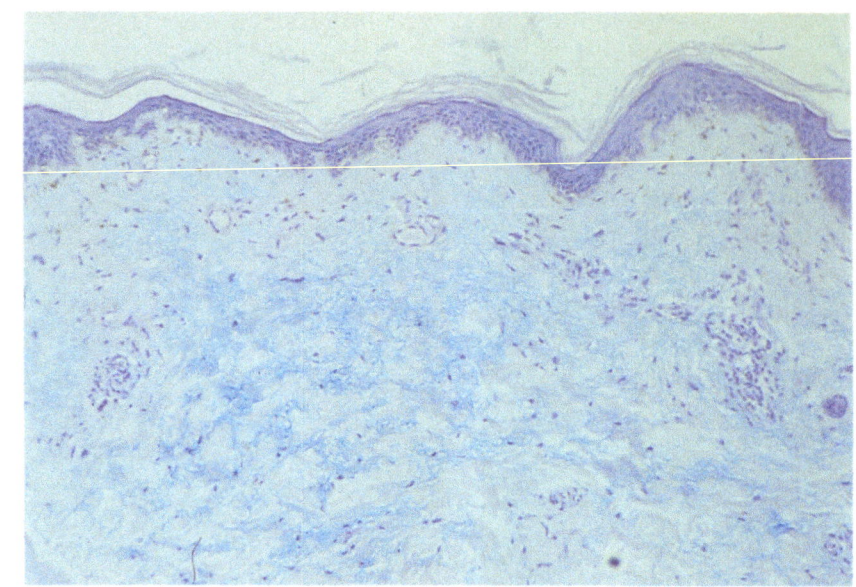

Plate 4 Histology of the skin in dermatomyositis showing mucin deposition in the dermis (stained with Alcian blue). (Courtesy of Dr N.P. Smith.)

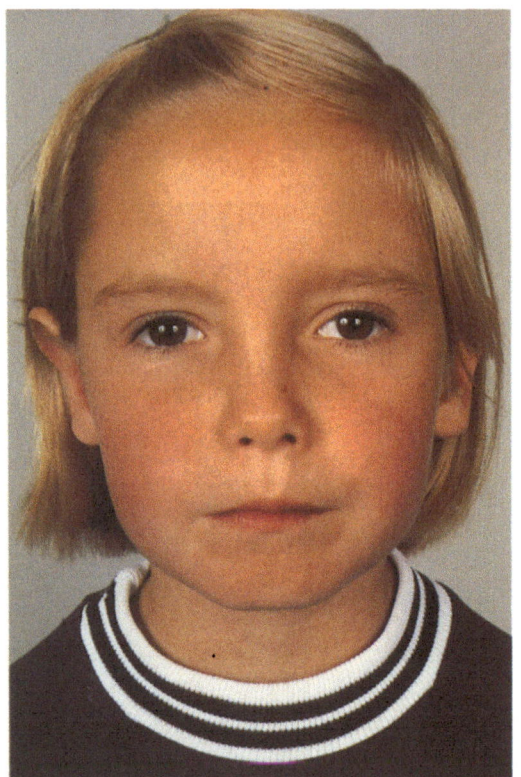

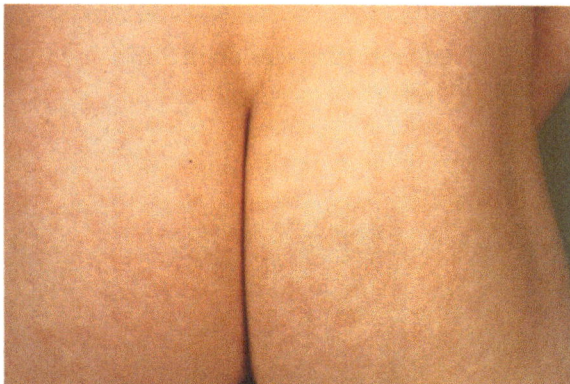

Plate 5 Erythema infectiosum: (a) cheek erythema – 'slapped cheeks'; (b) buttock erythema (note the reticulate 'chicken wire' pattern).

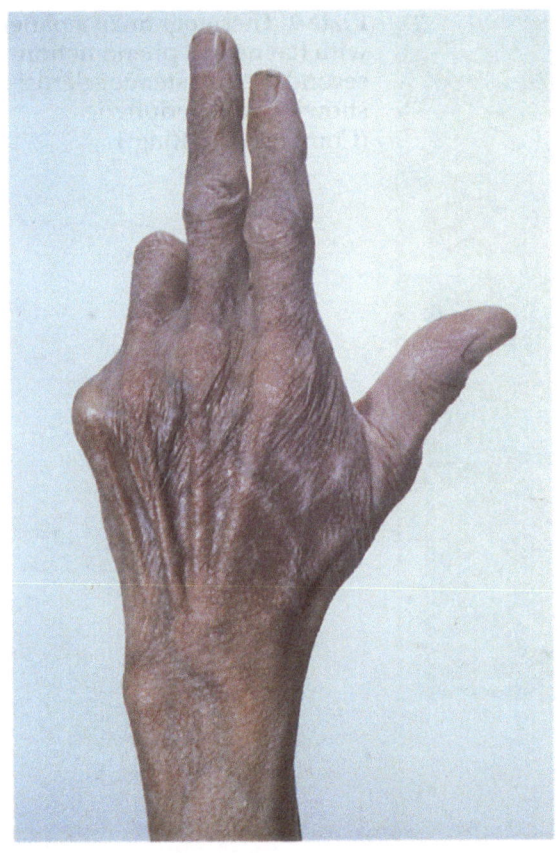

Plate 6 Haemochromatosis. Slatey grey-brown pigmentation affects light exposed areas and flexures.

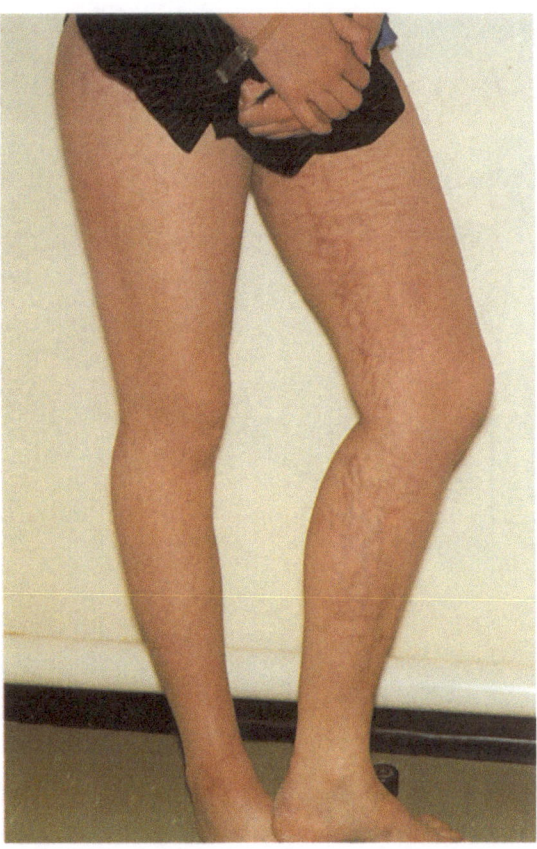

Plate 8 Striae due to excessive topical steroid therapy in childhood.

Plate 7 Sweet's syndrome – typical plum-coloured lesions.

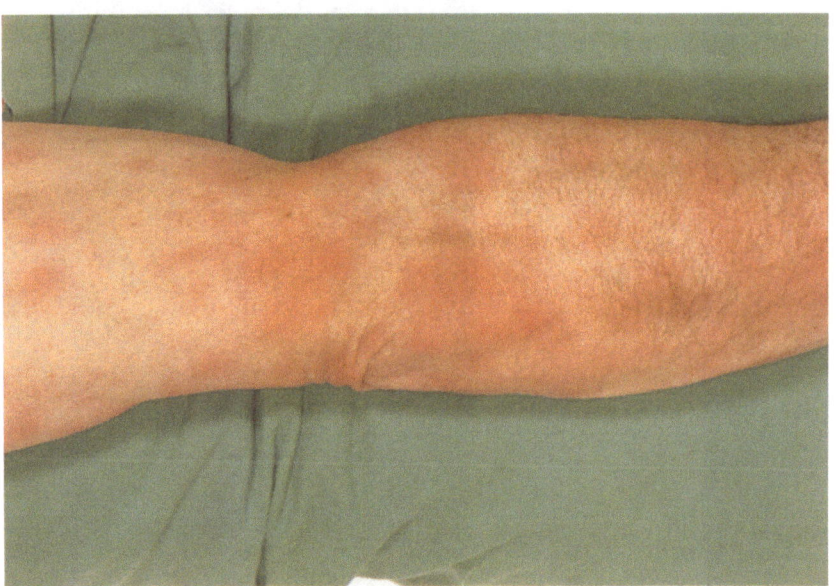

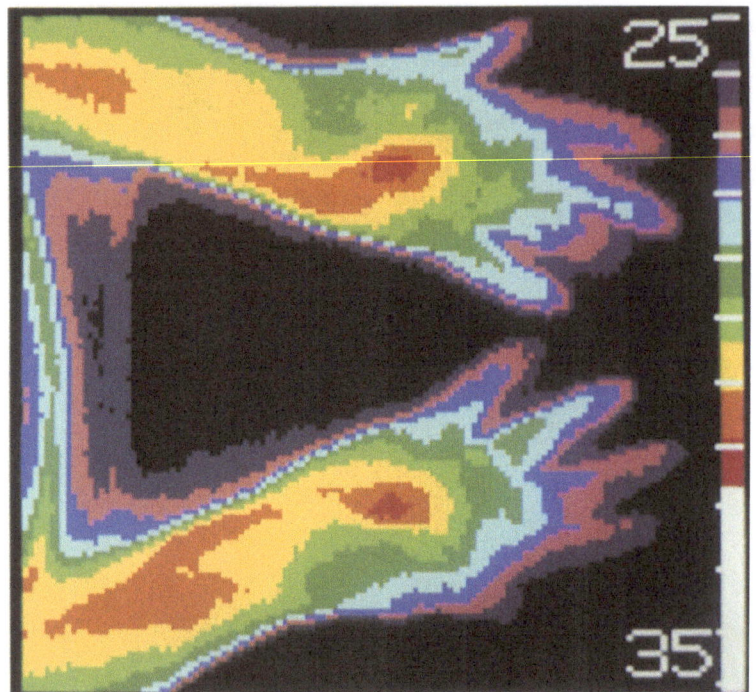

Plate 9 Thermogram of a patient with Raynaud's phenomenon secondary to systemic sclerosis showing cold peripheries. (Courtesy of F. Ring.)

Plate 10 Thermogram of normal hands. (Courtesy of F. Ring.)

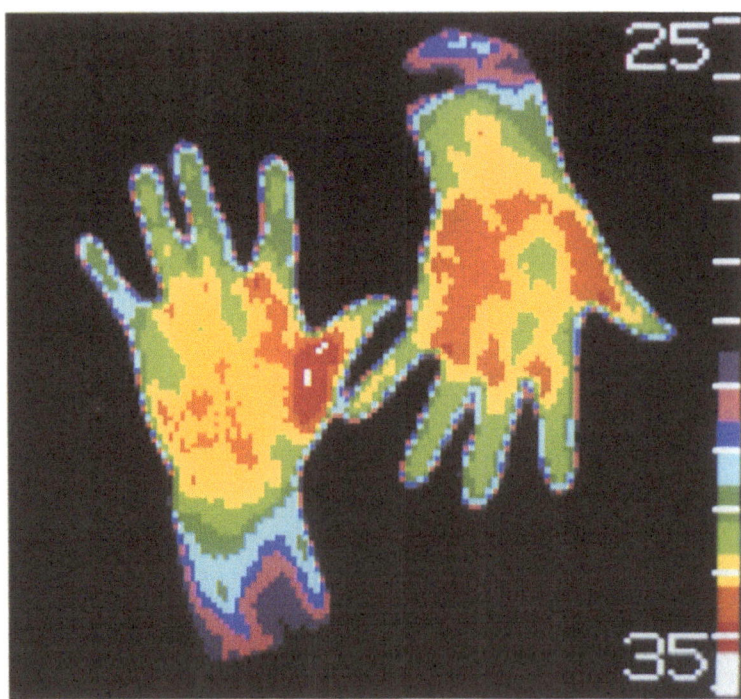

corticosteroid therapy. Nail involvement is common (Fig. 6.3) (80% in psoriatic arthritis; 35% in psoriasis alone) and may be the sole feature. Pitting is the commonest abnormality. Small deep pits of psoriasis should be distinguished from the shallow pits in atopic eczema. Onycholysis (increased separation of the free edge of the nail) is usually associated with subungual hyperkeratosis in distinction to other causes of onycholysis,

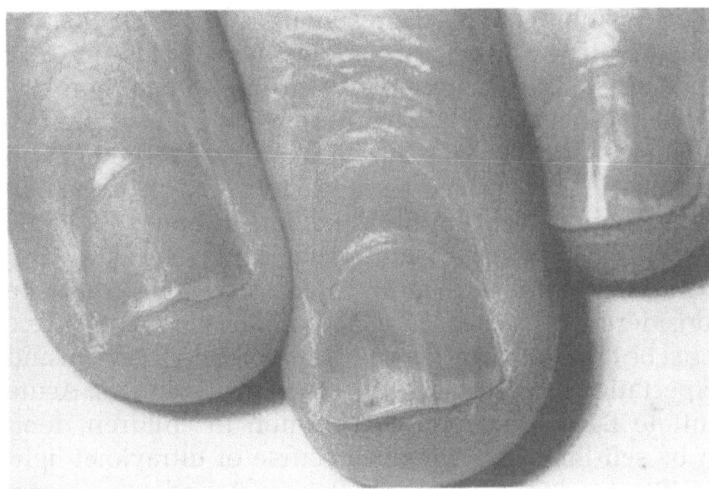

Fig. 6.3 Psoriatic nail involvement: (a) Onycholysis (separation of free edge of the nail) and salmon patch proximal to it. (b) Nail pitting.

(a)

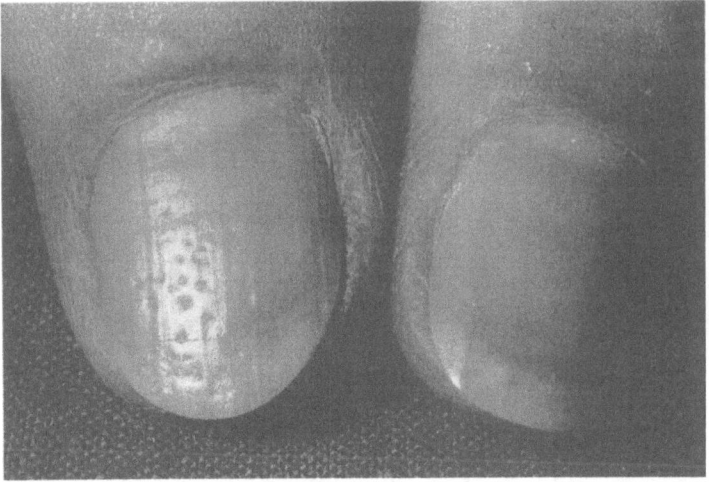

(b)

for example, thyrotoxicosis. Yellowish brown discoloration of the nail bed (salmon patch) is often seen proximal to the area of onycholysis. Ridging is not a diagnostic feature. Distal interphalangeal (DIP) joint disease is particularly associated with onycholysis (Fig. 6.4).

Certain patterns of arthritis have been described: the most common (60–70%) is asymmetrical oligoarthritis predominantly of large joints (Fig. 6.5a); symmetrical polyarthritis; predominant DIP involvement; axial involvement; arthritis mutilans (Fig. 6.5b). The 'sausage digit' is another typical presentation in which there is inflammation of the joint and surrounding tissues.

Psoriasis and rheumatoid arthritis are common diseases and may coexist. The presence of rheumatoid factor and subcutaneous nodules suggests rheumatoid disease. Pustular hyperkeratotic forms of psoriasis are indistinguishable from the cutaneous lesions of Reiter's disease (keratoderma blennorrhagica).

The treatment of skin and joint disease needs to be considered separately. Treatment of skin in psoriasis must be tailored to the needs of the individual patient and expectations of therapy vary between individuals. Acute guttate flares of psoriasis, common in children, tend to be self-limiting. A 6-week course of ultraviolet light (UVB), tar baths (such as Polytar®) and/or a cream containing extracts of coal tar such as Alphosyl® may hasten recovery. These measures may also be useful in

Fig. 6.4 Arthritis of distal interphalangeal (DIP) joints with severe nail changes, including onycholysis, pitting, subungual hyperkeratosis and paronychia.

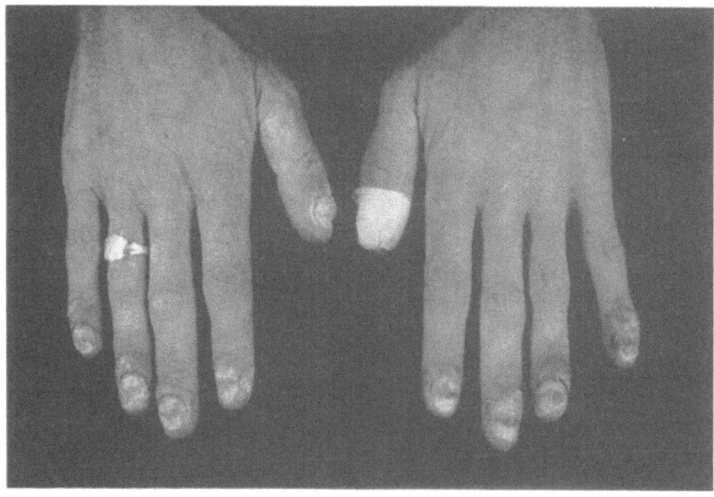

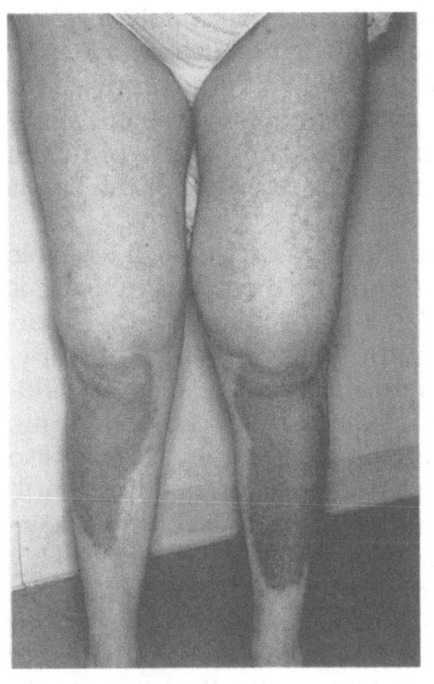

(a)

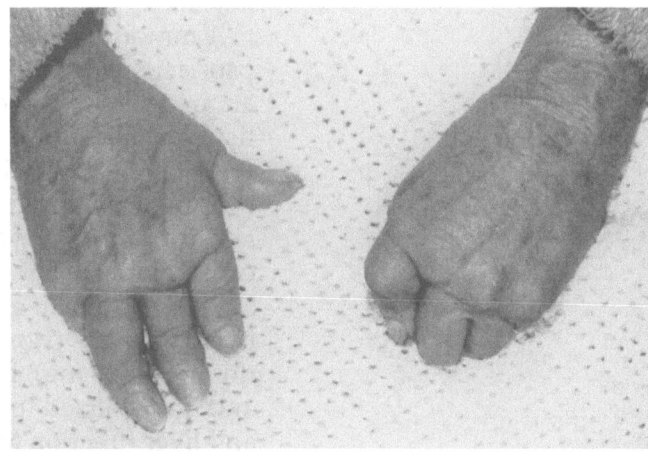

(b)

Fig. 6.5 Joint involvement in psoriatic arthritis. (a) Arthritis of knee with overlying psoriatic plaques. (b) Mutilating arthritis with telescoping digits due to small joint destruction ('main en lorgnette').

plaque psoriasis although often dithranol therapy is required. This is now available in a variety of cream and ointment bases (for example, Dithrocream®, Psoradrate cream®, Anthranol ointment® and in a wax stick base Antraderm®) which are more convenient to use in the patient's home than the traditional dithranol in Lassar's Paste BP. Individual tolerance to the irritant effects of dithranol varies widely. Initially a low concentration (for example, 0.1%) should be applied to the plaques, avoiding normal skin. Short-contact therapy (washing off the dithranol after $\frac{1}{2}$–2 hours) is more convenient than leaving the preparation on overnight, although somewhat less effective. The patient should be warned of mild irritation and staining, both of skin and clothes. Patients with more resistant plaque psoriasis require increasing concentrations of dithranol in Lassar's Paste either as a day case or admitted to a specialist dermatology unit. Dithranol should not be used on the face or flexures. Flexural psoriasis usually responds to dilute preparations of refined coal tar (for example, coal tar and salicylic acid ointment BP) or a dilute corticosteroid with tar (for example, Tarcortin cream® or Betnovate RD ung® with 5% liquor picis carbonis). Systemic corticosteroids should never be used and the use of potent topical corticosteroids should be reserved for the hands and feet.

A minority of patients with very extensive or unstable psoriasis will require second-line therapy. Etretinate is an aromatic retinoid related to vitamin A which is particularly effective in conjunction with topical therapy, UVB or PUVA. It is teratogenic, and women of child-bearing age should use adequate contraception during, and for at least 2 years following, therapy. It may also cause elevation of serum triglycerides and cholesterol. Several cytotoxic and immunosuppressive drugs have been used in psoriasis. Methotrexate, in low weekly dosage (5–15 mg), is particularly useful in erythrodermic and generalized pustular psoriasis. Full blood count and liver function tests should be checked regularly and most dermatologists carry out routine liver biopsies in younger patients on long term therapy. PUVA (psoralen plus UVA) is of value in recalcitrant hand and foot psoriasis and in many individuals with widespread disease, particularly when used in conjunction with etretinate ('Re PUVA'). It is potentially carcinogenic to the skin and long term PUVA should be reserved, if possible, for older patients.

Treatment of joint disease varies according to the pattern of involvement. Asymmetrical involvement of large joints tends to be more benign. Symptomatic treatment with non-steroidal anti-inflammatory drugs (NSAIDs), occasional use of intra-articular steroid injection and physiotherapy is usually adequate. Severe arthritis may require disease-modifying therapy such as azathioprine, or methotrexate if there is significant skin disease. Recent studies suggest that etretinate is also beneficial in joint disease. Antimalarials are contraindicated as they may exacerbate skin disease.

6.3 REITER'S DISEASE

Classically a triad of urethritis, conjunctivitis and arthritis which can be precipitated by multiple infective triggers predominantly involving the gastrointestinal and genitourinary tract. It can occur at any age, but typically in young males. Mucocutaneous involvement is often an early feature and characteristically transient and painless. Shallow buccal erosions are common often with an erythematous margin. Circinate balanitis occurs on the glans and shaft of the penis in approximately 30% of patients (Fig. 6.6). In the circumcised, lesions remain discrete and crusted, whilst in the uncircumcised they frequently coalesce and remain moist. The term keratoderma blennorrhagica (Fig. 6.7) describes hyperkeratotic pustules occurring in 15% predominantly on the soles and palms. These lesions are indistinguishable from some variants of psoriasis and may coalesce to form large plaques. Rarely, lesions occur elsewhere such as scrotum, trunk and scalp. Nail dystrophy may occur with subungual hyperkeratosis.

Arthritis is predominantly asymmetrical and involves the large joints especially the knees. Sacroiliitis, which is often asymmetrical (Fig. 6.8) and spondylitis are strongly linked with HLA B27. Enthesopathy is prominent. Conjunctivitis or iritis may present as a 'red eye' (Fig. 6.9).

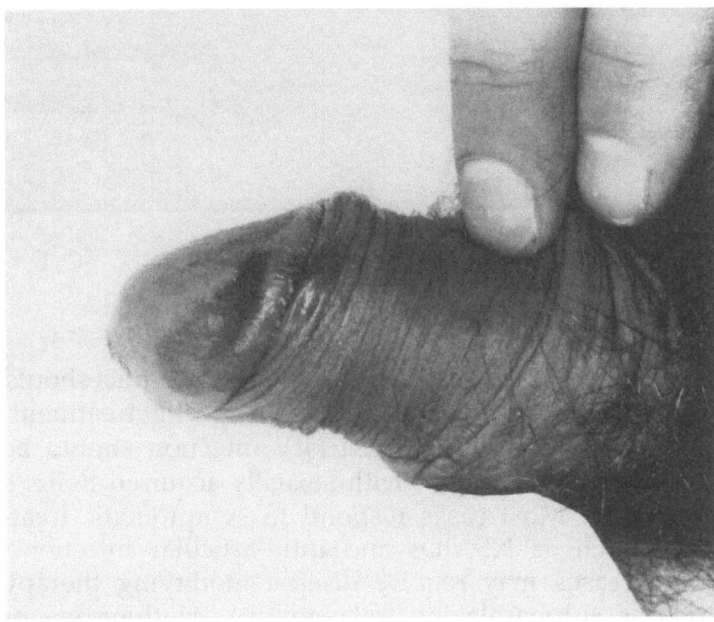

Fig. 6.6 Circinate balanitis of the glans penis.

Fig. 6.7 Keratoderma blennorrhagica. Hyperkeratotic lesions on the fingers of a young man with Reiter's disease.

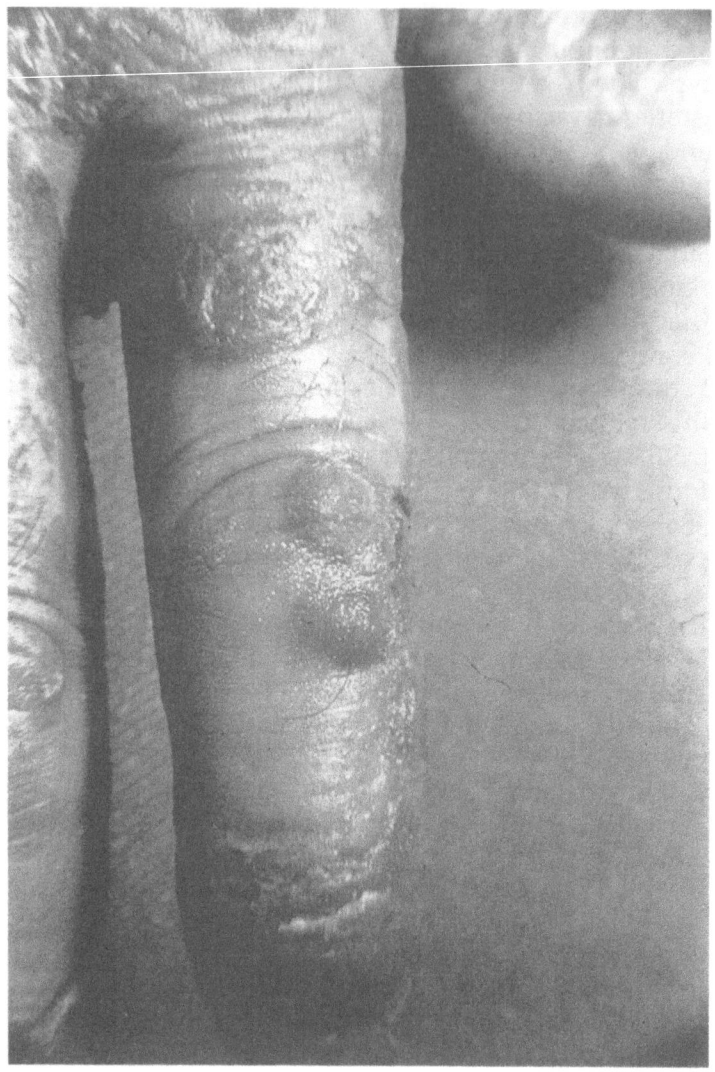

6.3.1 Management

Infection of the urogenital or gastrointestinal tract should be investigated since this may need specific treatment. The possibility of associated HIV infection should be considered in a patient with sexually acquired Reiter's syndrome. Most cases respond to symptomatic treatment such as NSAIDs and intra-articular injections; severe cases may require disease modifying therapy such as sulphasalazine (salazopyrin), azathioprine or

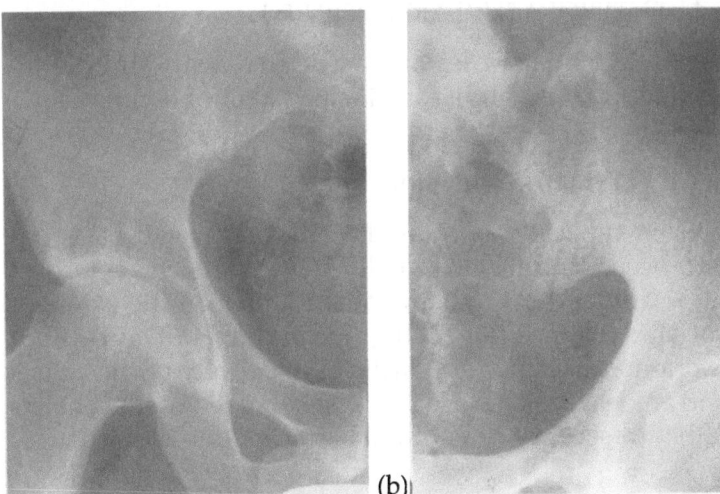

(a) (b)

Fig. 6.8 Sacroiliitis. (a) early stages, (b) late stages showing obliteration of the joints.

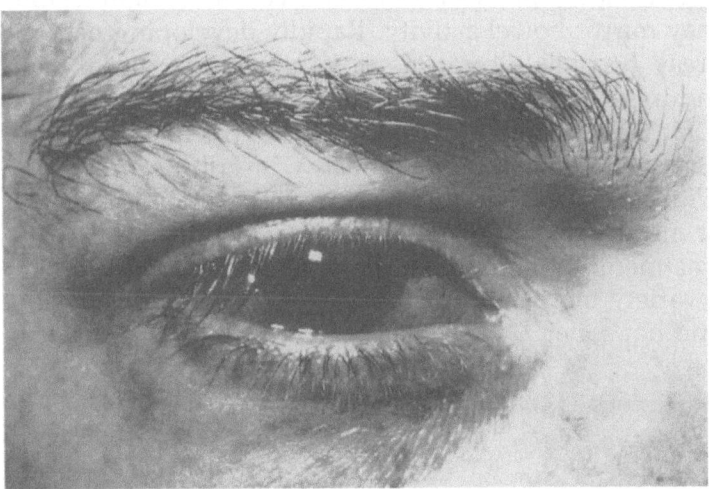

Fig. 6.9 'Red eye' due to iritis in Reiter's disease.

methotrexate. Skin disease is often transient: severe cases require topical steroids, tetracycline, systemic retinoids and/or PUVA.

6.3.2 Course and prognosis

The initial attack generally settles but the majority relapse and continue to have intermittent or persistent disease. Skin and mucous membrane involvement may follow a different course from that of the joints.

6.4   ENTEROPATHIC ARTHROPATHY

Characteristic skin lesions associated with chronic inflammatory bowel disease include the following.

6.4.1   Erythema nodosum

This is typically associated with Crohn's disease but also occurs in ulcerative colitis (UC). It is characterized by warm tender erythematous nodules on the extensor surfaces of limbs (Fig. 6.10), healing without scarring. It is often associated with arthritis especially of the wrists and ankles. Patients are often febrile. Treatment consists of bed rest and non-steroidal anti-inflammatory drugs.

6.4.2   Pyoderma gangrenosum

This is classically seen in ulcerative colitis. Skin lesions may mirror bowel activity. Rapidly developing necrotic areas become ulcerated, sloughing and painful with indurated violaceous and undermined margins (Fig. 6.11a). The trunk, legs, buttocks are principally affected. Lesions may heal spontaneously with cribriform scarring (Fig. 6.11b). Severe cases often require systemic steroids, or intralesional steroids, but will sometimes respond to treatment of the cause. Individual cases may respond to a variety of agents, including clofazimine, minocycline and dapsone.

Fig. 6.10   Erythema nodosum of lower leg showing shiny infiltrated nodules and oedema.

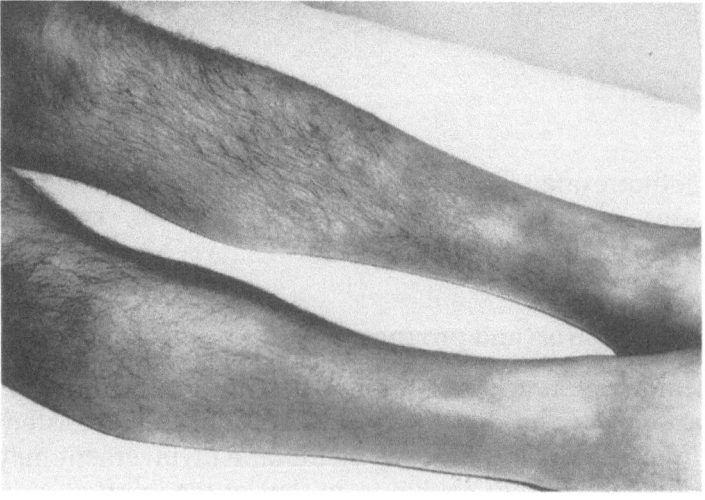

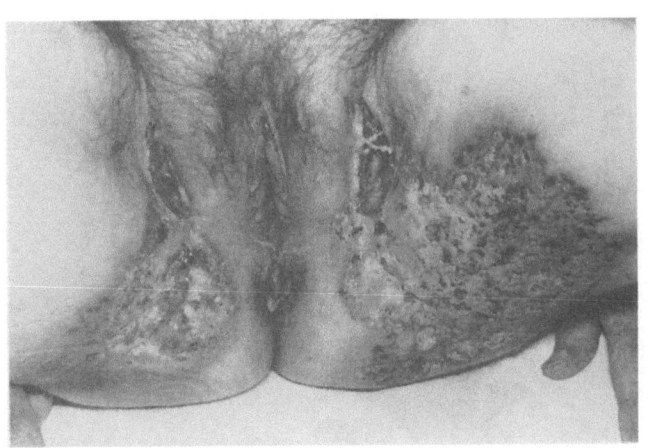
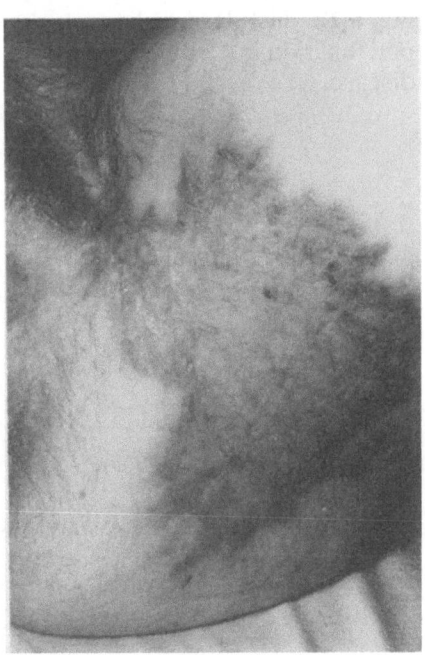

(a)   (b)

Fig. 6.11   Pyoderma gangrenosum associated with Crohn's disease. (a) Deep sloughing ulcer with characteristic undermined margin. (b) Healed ulcer with cribriform scarring.

6.4.3   Aphthous mucous membrane ulceration

This is common especially in Crohn's disease. Other cutaneous manifestations of Crohn's include sinuses and fistulae (Fig. 6.12) and granulomatous cheilitis (Fig. 6.13).

Peripheral joint involvement predominantly affects large joints and reflects bowel activity. Cutaneous and joint manifestations respond to disease modifying therapy such as sulphasalazine. A proportion have sacroiliitis identical to ankylosing spondylitis and similarly associated with HLA B27. Treatment is with NSAIDS and active physiotherapy.

6.4.4   Jejunoileal bypass surgery

Some 20% of patients who receive bypass surgery for morbid obesity develop skin and joint lesions. The aetiology is thought to be immune complex mediated and antibody to intestinal organisms has been detected in lesions. Skin lesions are macules, affecting the extensor

Fig. 6.12 Fistulae involving perianal skin in Crohn's disease.

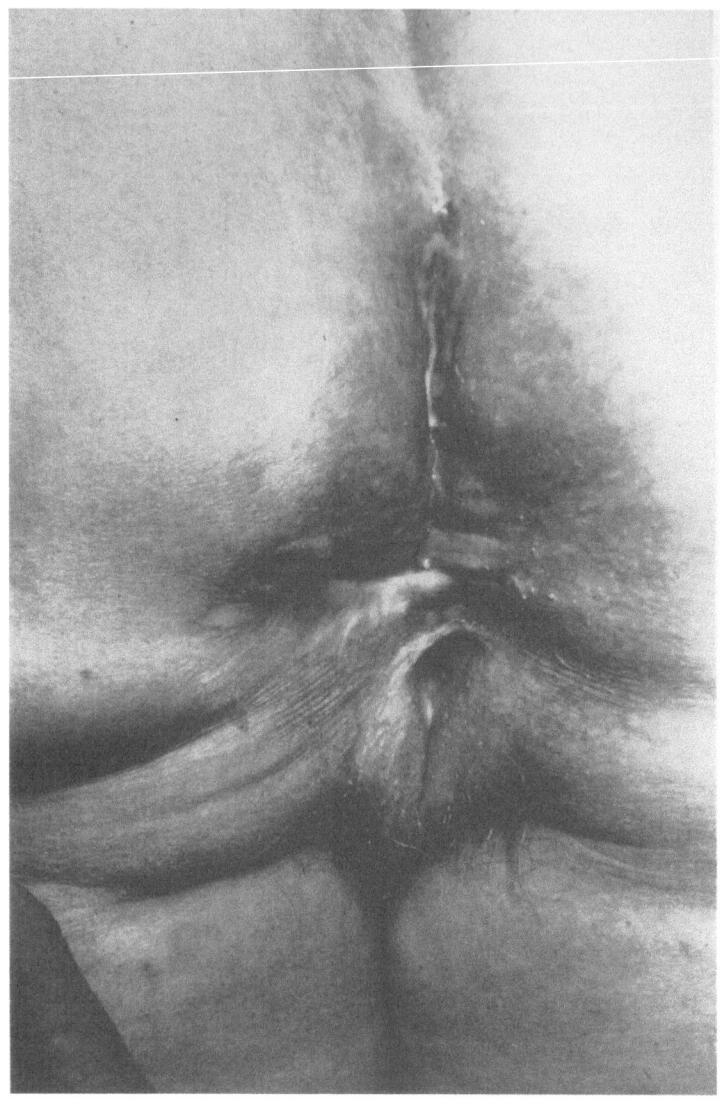

surfaces of the limbs, buttocks and lower abdomen, which may become tender pustules (Figs 6.14a and 6.14b) followed by desquamation. Histology shows leucocyto-clastic vasculitis (Fig. 6.14c). Erythema nodosum may occur. Arthralgia or symmetrical polyarthritis typically affects knees, metacarpophalangeal joints, wrists and shoulders. The axial skeleton is spared. Pleurisy, peri-carditis and a mesangial glomerulonephritis have been reported. Mild cases respond to NSAIDS. More severe

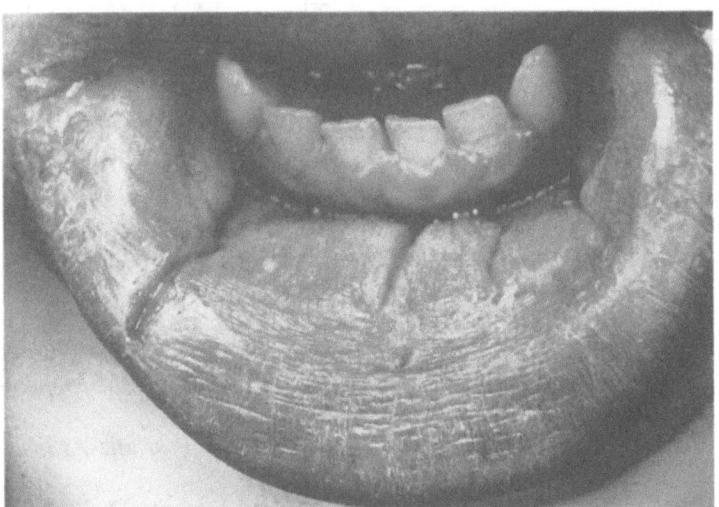

Fig. 6.13 Cheilitis showing swollen rugose lip with fissuring in Crohn's disease.

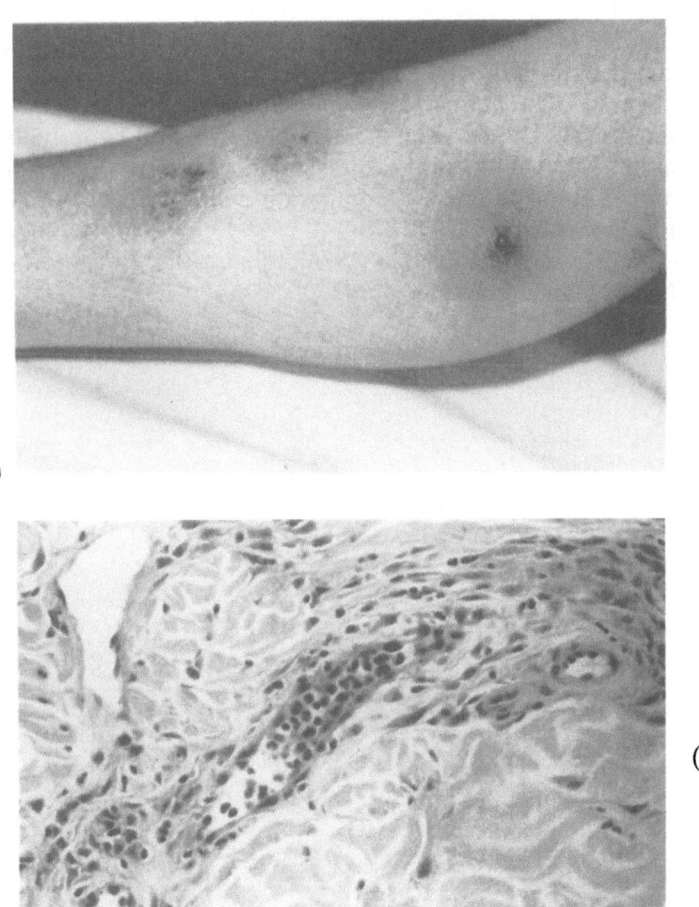

(a)

(c)

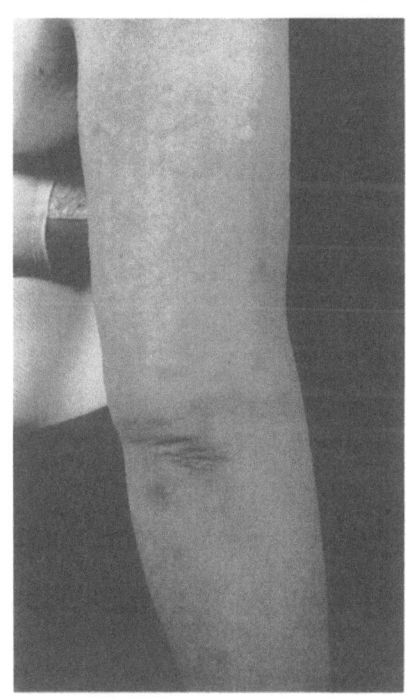

(b)

Fig. 6.14 (a) and (b) Pustular lesions on limbs following small bowel bypass surgery. (c) Histology showing small vessel vasculitis (Courtesy of Dr C. T. C. Kennedy.)

forms may require antibiotics, dapsone, or even systemic steroids. Intractable cases may require bypass reversal.

BIBLIOGRAPHY

Baden, H. P. (ed.) (1984) *The Chemotherapy of Psoriasis*. Pergamon Press, Oxford.

Fox, R., Calin, A., Gerbo, R. C. and Gibson, D. (1979) The chronicity of symptoms and disability in Reiter's syndrome: an analysis of 131 consecutive patients. *Annals of Internal Medicine* **91**, 190–8.

Gerber, L. H. and Espinoza, L. R. (1985) *Psoriatic Arthritis*. Grune and Stratton, New York.

Greenstein, A. J., Janowitz, H. D. and Sachar, D. B. (1976) The extraintestinal complications of Crohn's disease and ulcerative colitis: a study of 200 patients. *Medicine* **55**, 401–11.

Moll, J. M. H. (1980) *Ankylosing Spondylitis*. Churchill Livingstone, Edinburgh.

McEwan, C., Di Tata, D., Lingg, C., Porini, A., Good, A. and Rankin, T. (1971) Ankylosing spondylitis and spondylitis accompanying ulcerative colitis, regional enteritis, psoriasis and Reiter's disease: a comparative study. *Arthritis and Rheumatism*, **14**, 291–318.

Wright, V., Moll, J. M. H. (1976) *Seronegative Polyarthritis*. North-Holland, Amsterdam.

CHAPTER SEVEN

The skin in rheumatoid arthritis

The skin does not bear the brunt of disease in rheumatoid arthritis (RA) unlike other connective tissue disorders. However, skin manifestations reflect the systemic nature of RA or its association with other autoimmune disorders. Cutaneous drug effects are common (see Chapter 10).

7.1 RHEUMATOID NODULES

Subcutaneous nodules are a specific manifestation of RA. They occur in approximately 30% and are associated with seropositivity for rheumatoid factor and other extra-articular manifestations. They vary in size up to several centimetres and are found over extensor surfaces, often related to bony prominences, and probably reflect tissue trauma. The precise features determining nodule formation are unknown but local pressure plays an important part and characteristic sites are the elbow, especially the proximal ulna and within olecranon bursae, the knuckles, the sacrum (Fig. 7.1) and sometimes on the ear and over the occiput in the bedbound patient. Sacral nodules in particular may break down and form persistent troublesome ulcers. Methotrexate therapy may stimulate nodule formation in RA. Histology of nodules is characteristic (Fig. 7.2). In a well formed nodule there is a central area of necrosis ringed by palisading fibroblasts.

While some patients have large single rather rubbery nodules, often over the elbow, which show little change in size over months or years, others develop crops of multiple small nodules which are often intracutaneous and perforate the epidermis. These appear and disappear more rapidly than large nodules and are associ-

Fig. 7.1 Rheumatoid nodules: (a) Situated over metacarpophalangeal joints. (b) Over extensor surface of the forearm and in an olecranon bursa. (c) Over the knees. (d) On the sacrum.

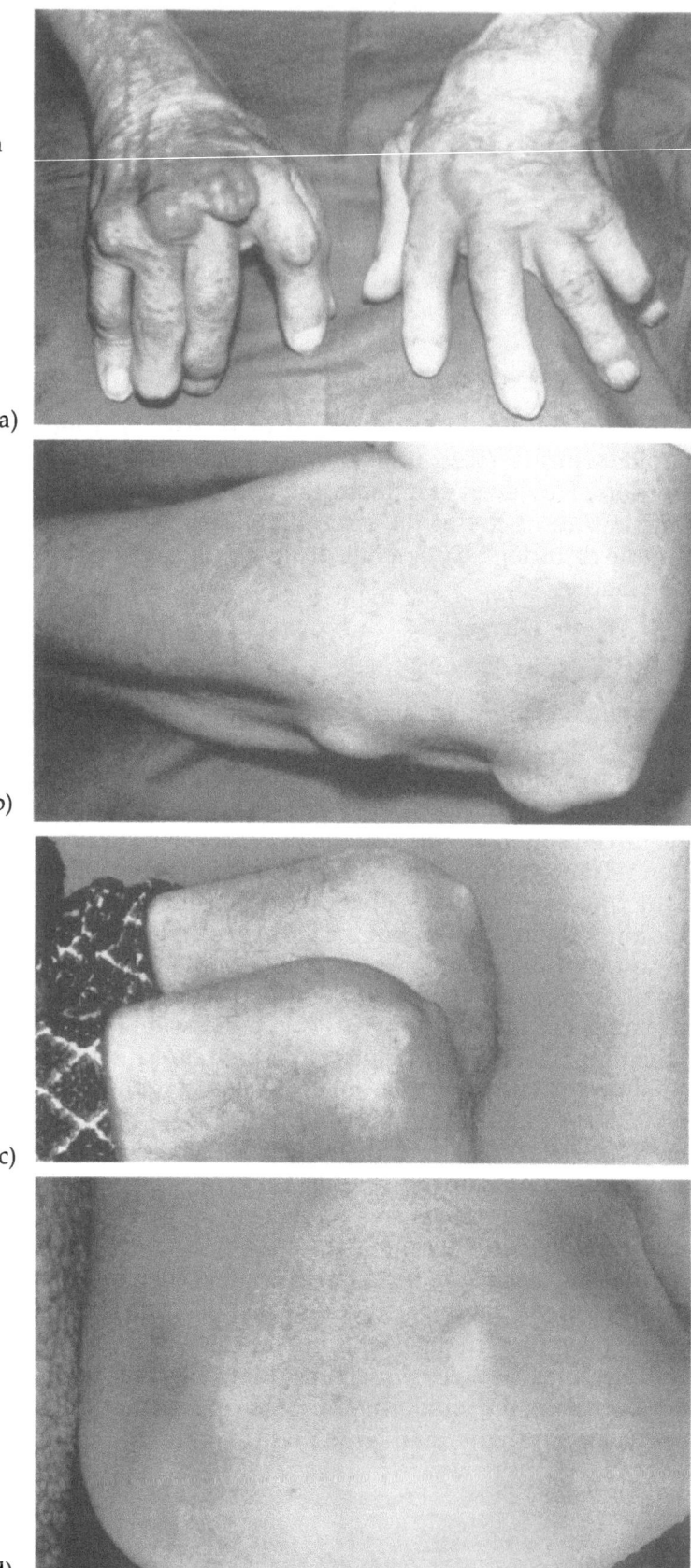

(a)

(b)

(c)

(d)

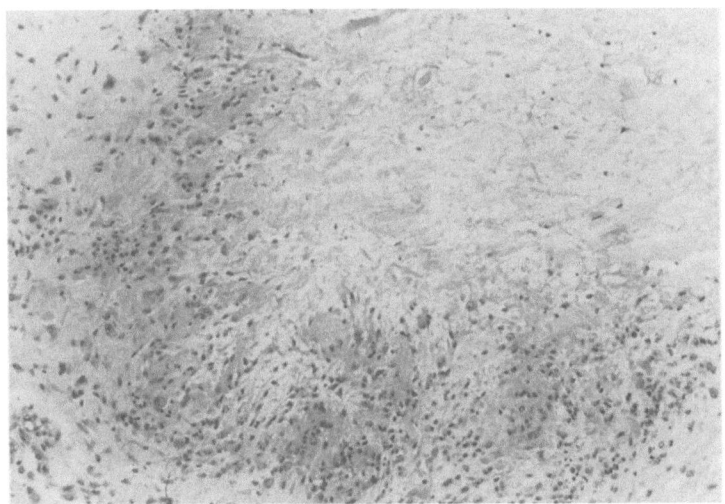

Fig. 7.2 Histology of part of a rheumatoid nodule showing central fibrinoid necrosis surrounded by palisading fibroblasts. (Courtesy of Dr T. I. Macleod.)

ated with active systemic features of rheumatoid disease such as vasculitis. Superficial nodules may mimic perforating lesions of granuloma annulare. These are intracutaneous and are not necessarily associated with other disease.

Nodules over pressure points need to be differentiated from xanthomata, which usually have a yellow tinge and are associated with increased plasma levels of lipoproteins and cholesterol, and tophi which are associated with elevated levels of uric acid and from which urate crystals can be aspirated. Benign nodules with histology similar to rheumatoid nodules occasionally develop on the pretibial region, feet and scalp of otherwise normal healthy children. These nodules resolve spontaneously.

Firm, painless subcutaneous bands in the axillary line have been described in patients with nodular rheumatoid disease.

7.2 VASCULITIS

Vasculitis is a feature of active systemic disease and may be precipitated by corticosteroid therapy. Any vessel or a combination of vessels can be involved; the size and site determining the clinical manifestations and prognosis. Most commonly involvement is restricted to small, digital arterioles, resulting in periungual and nailfold infarcts (Fig. 7.3). Less frequently systemic leucocytoclastic vasculitis occurs. This may be limited to a leucocytoclastic vasculitis affecting the skin (where it

Fig. 7.3   (a) and (b) Digital
vasculitis in rheumatoid disease.
(7.3b Courtesy of Dr Allan St J.
Dixon.)

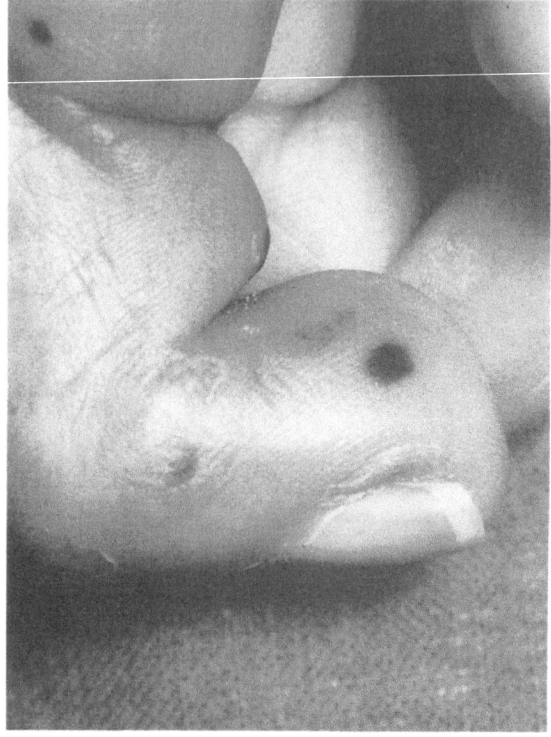

(a)

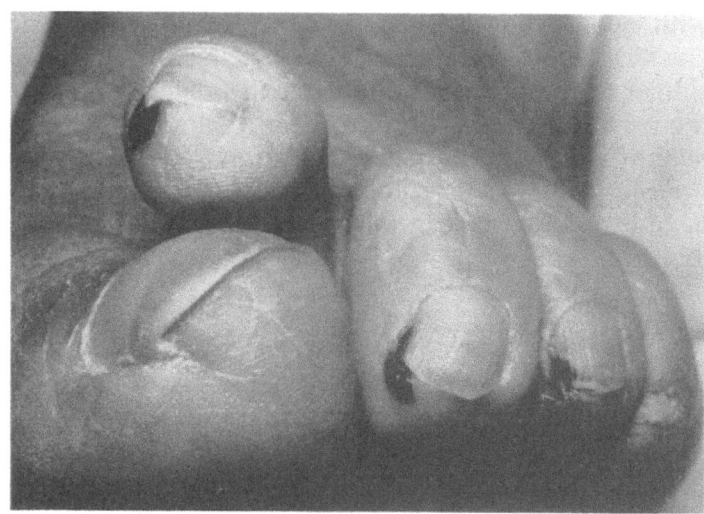

(b)

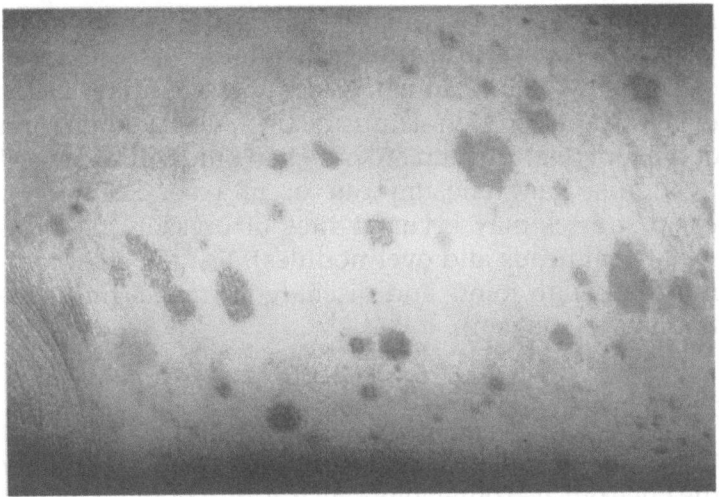

Fig. 7.4 Palpable purpura due to leukocytoclastic vasculitis in the dermis.

may present as an urticarial vasculitis) (Fig. 7.4) and kidneys producing microscopic haematuria and sometimes mild proteinuria, and carries a good prognosis. Conversely, involvement of medium sized and small arteries resembling PAN (see Chapter 5) represents a serious and potentially fatal complication.

7.3 CUTANEOUS ULCERATION

Cutaneous ulceration, particularly affecting the lower legs, is common and is multifactorial. Immobility and

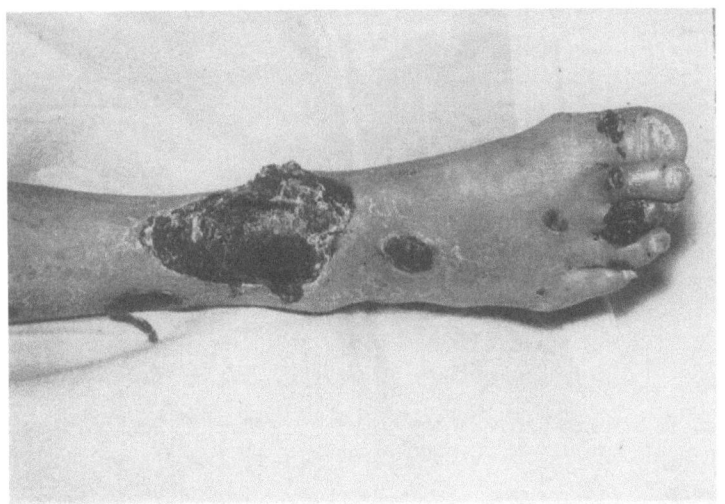

Fig. 7.5 Vasculitic ulcers. Typical features are rapid development, punched-out appearance and sites on the dorsum of the foot and anterior ankle.

involvement of lower limb joints, especially the ankle joint, predispose to chronic gravitational ulcers which often follow skin trauma. In contrast vasculitic ulcers develop rapidly, often at unusual sites such as the dorsum of the foot (Fig. 7.5) and are punched out. Rarely, typical pyoderma gangrenosum can occur (see Chapter 6). Deep sinuses may occur at sites of pressure (such as metatarsal heads and over nodules). Fistulae may communicate with joints and discharge synovial fluid (fistulous rheumatism).

7.4 JOINT RUPTURE

Occasionally inflamed joints rupture, most commonly the knee but also other joints such as the shoulder, elbow and wrist. Rupture of the knee joint with leakage of synovial fluid into the fascial planes can simulate a deep venous thrombosis and a correct diagnosis is required

Fig. 7.6 Ruptured shoulder showing ecchymoses in the upper arm.

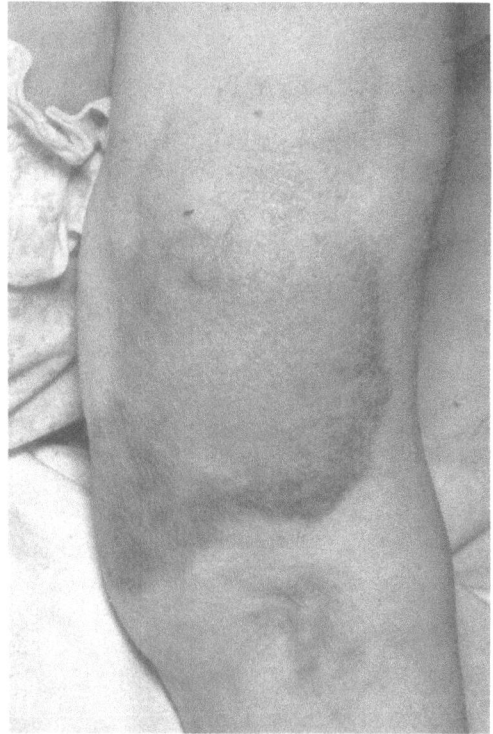

to avoid inappropriate therapy with anticoagulants. Past history of arthritis, inflammation of the associated joint and the presence of bruising (crescent sign) due to haemorrhage into the tissues are important features. An arthrogram confirms the diagnosis.

7.5 OTHER CUTANEOUS MANIFESTATIONS

There is thinning of the skin which is often pale, translucent and atrophic especially on the hands and feet. This may be exacerbated by corticosteroid therapy. Early on in the course of the disease the fingers may be oedematous and stiff resembling sclerodactyly. Later, palmar erythema (Fig. 7.7) is a frequent feature. Localized hyperpigmentation may be found overlying acutely inflamed joints while diffuse pigmentation may develop in patients with active systemic disease and has been particularly associated with Felty's syndrome. Raynaud's phenomenon may occur and in some patients it indicates the development of carpal tunnel compression. Hyperkeratosis occurs over weight-bearing areas especially over metatarsal heads. The development of Sjögren's syndrome is associated with dryness of the skin and mucous membranes. Vitiligo is an associated autoimmune manifestation and diffuse alopecia may also occur. Alopecia areata is another autoimmune disorder associated with rheumatoid disease.

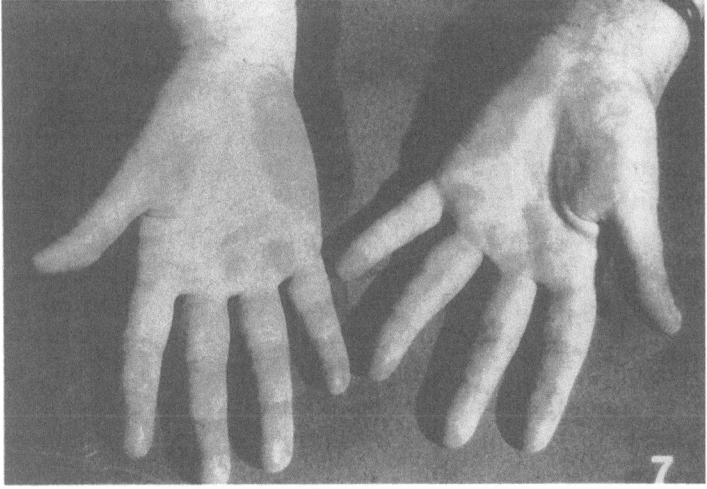

Fig. 7.7 Palmar erythema in a patient with RA.

Fig. 7.8 Dusky
hyperpigmentation overlying
inflamed joints in rheumatoid
arthritis. (Courtesy of Dr Allan
St John Dixon.)

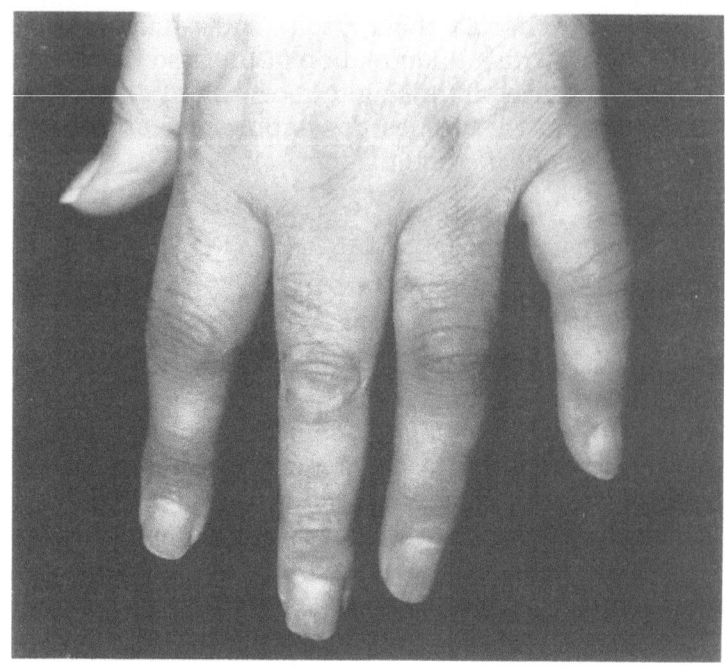

7.6   SEPTIC ARTHRITIS

Rheumatoid patients are particularly susceptible to septic joints particularly due to staphylococcus (see Chapter 8). This is an important differential diagnosis of exacerbation of joint disease particularly in a single joint since systemic manifestations of infection are frequently masked. Symptoms and signs are also masked in individuals on corticosteroid therapy.

7.7   MANAGEMENT

Important preventive measures to reduce skin trauma include appropriate footwear, measures to increase mobility and chiropody.

The management of leg ulcers in RA includes bedrest and treatment of underlying disease including anaemia; controlling exudation and encouraging granulation of clean ulcers with occlusive dressings. Vasculitic ulcers are reported to respond to disease modifying therapy such as methotrexate or cyclophosphamide.

Major vessel vasculitis justifies the aggressive use of cytotoxic drugs such as cyclophosphamide. Less serious forms of vasculitis and nodules respond to conventional disease modifying agents such as gold or D-penicillamine. Surgical removal of nodules can lead to persisting sinuses or fistulae. They may, however, respond to intralesional corticosteroids.

BIBLIOGRAPHY

Collins, D. H. (1937) The subcutaneous nodule of rheumatoid arthritis. *Journal of Pathology and Bacteriology*, **45**, 97–117.
Gardner, D. L. (1972) *The Pathology of Rheumatoid Arthritis*. Edward Arnold, London.
Scott, D. G. I., Bacon, P. A. and Tribe, C. R. (1981) Systemic rheumatoid vasculitis: a clinical and laboratory study of 50 cases. *Medicine*, **60**, 285–97.

CHAPTER EIGHT

Infections

Various organisms affect both skin and joints, either by direct infection or via immunological mechanisms. The pattern of skin involvement is often characteristic and may aid diagnosis. Organisms of low infectivity such as fungi may induce lesions in immunocompromised patients.

8.1 BACTERIAL INFECTIONS

8.1.1 Septic arthritis

Those at risk from septic arthritis are people with pre-existing joint disease, especially rheumatoid arthritis, the elderly, the chronically debilitated and the immuno-suppressed individual. Staphylococci are the commonest causative agent but Gram negative infections have become increasingly prevalent especially in the elderly and immunologically compromised.

The infected joint usually arises from a bacteraemia though frequently a primary septic focus is not found. Typically the presentation is with acute onset of pain and swelling in a single large joint, particularly the knee although any joint may be involved and polyarticular involvement is seen. The overlying skin may be warm and erythematous. Often symptoms and signs are not dramatic especially in a patient with rheumatoid arthritis when constitutional signs of infection may be minimal, particularly if the patient is taking corticosteroids.

Aspiration of pus from the joint with identification of bacteria in Gram staining and subsequent culture confirms the diagnosis. Prompt treatment is essential to avoid destruction and deformity of the joint and to safeguard the patient since delayed diagnosis is associated with high mortality. Treatment consists of appropriate antibiotics in effective doses given for at least 8 weeks

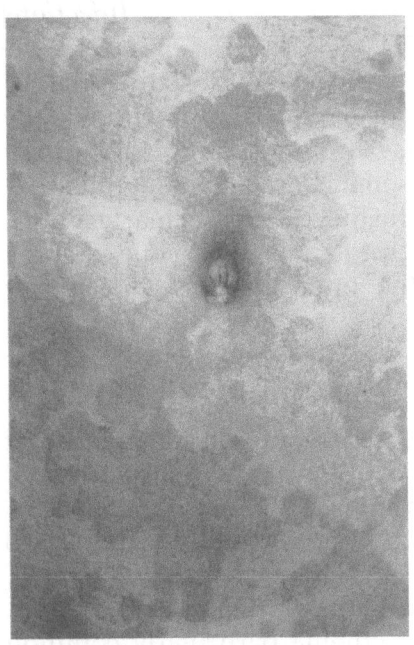

(a)

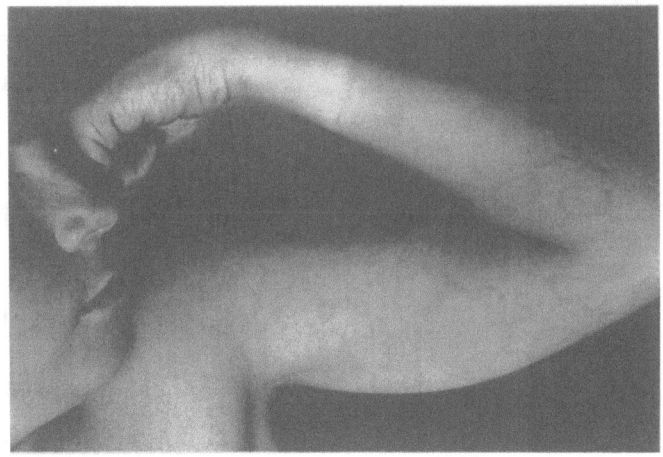

(b)

Fig. 8.1 (a), (b), (c), (d)
Erythema marginatum. A
transient erythema (lasting at
most 2–3 days) which may
occur at any stage of the
disease, including relapse.
Reddish annular lesions may
enlarge to form large figurate
patches within hours. Lesions
may recur and are most
noticeable in the afternoon.
(Fig. 8.1a, Courtesy of Dr
E. Pascual; Figs 8.1b, c, d
Courtesy of Prof E. G.
Bywaters.)

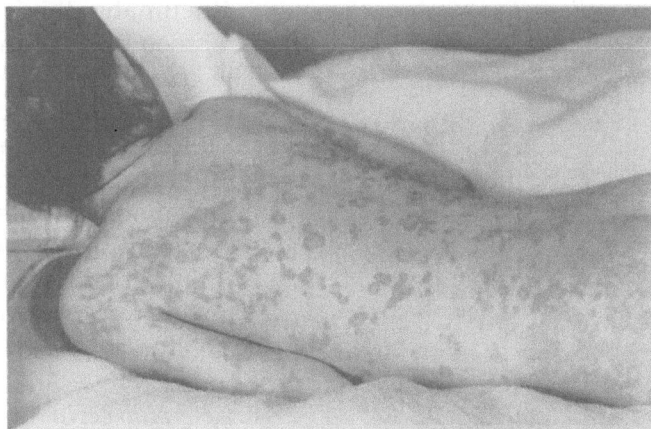

(c)

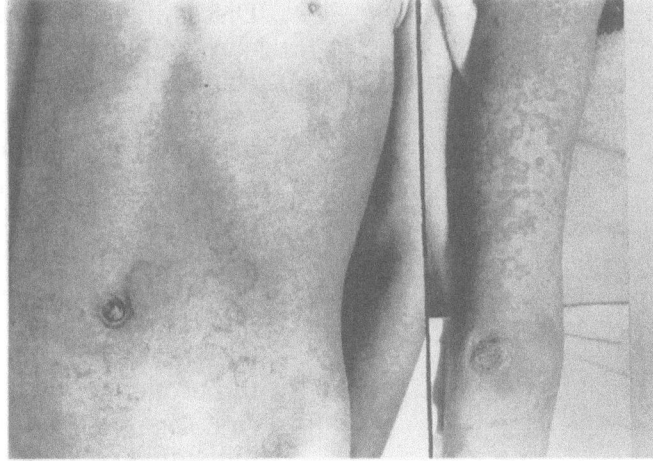

(d)

and drainage is usually achieved by closed needle aspiration to relieve intra-articular pressure and potentially damaging enzymes released from polymorphs. The joint should be mobilized as soon as symptoms permit.

Infection of a joint prosthesis is particularly grave. Although drainage and prolonged antibiotic therapy can sometimes be effective often it becomes necessary to remove the prosthesis.

8.1.2 Streptococcal infections

Beta-haemolytic streptococci are an important cause of erythema nodosum (see Chapter 6) and rarely a cause of Henoch–Schönlein purpura (see Chapter 5).

Rheumatic fever is an immunological reaction to streptococci. It is increasingly rare in Western society. The characteristic skin lesion is erythema marginatum, an evanescent annular erythema particularly common in children (Fig. 8.1a, b, c, d). A flitting arthritis is typical with erythema overlying affected joints. Subcutaneous nodules and papules may develop over bony prominences. Joint involvement predominates in adults, a deforming arthritis (Jaccoud's) is rare and resembles that seen in systemic lupus erythematosus (see Fig. 3.11, page 40).

8.1.3 *Neisseria*

Gonococcal

Disseminated gonococcal infection occurs primarily in chronic female carriers. An initial bacteraemic state is characterized by a migratory arthritis, sometimes accompanied by typical skin lesions (Fig. 8.2). These occur in small crops composed of greyish vesicles later forming haemorrhagic blisters or pustules. Subsequently a septic monoarthritis or oligoarthritis may follow, characteristically accompanied by tenosynovitis especially of the hands and wrists. Occasionally organisms can be isolated from blood cultures, skin lesions, and joints. However, bacteriological confirmation is usually obtained from the urogenital tract. Treatment follows the same principles as for other forms of septic arthritis. However, disseminated gonococcal infection is very sensitive to penicillin. The most widely used regimen is penicillin G

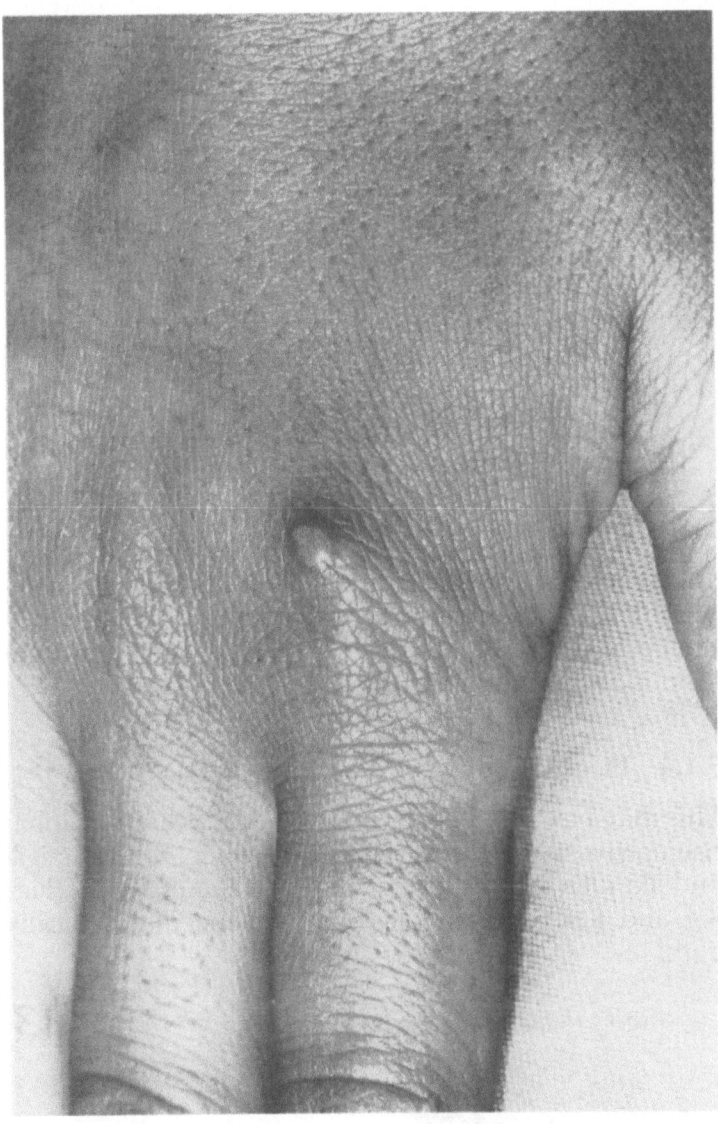

Fig. 8.2 Gonococcal pustule. Lesions are most commonly found on the fingers.

10 million units intravenously until symptoms subside followed by ampicillin for 10 days.

Neisseria meningitidis

Similar, but more widespread haemorrhagic pustules occur in *N. meningitidis* bacteraemia (Fig. 8.3), which may be accompanied by a flitting arthritis particularly of the knees. Most cases occur in young children although

Fig. 8.3 Haemorrhagic lesions in bacteraemia due to *Neisseria meningitidis*. Scattered petechial areas of variable size may be associated with large plaques of haemorrhagic gangrene.

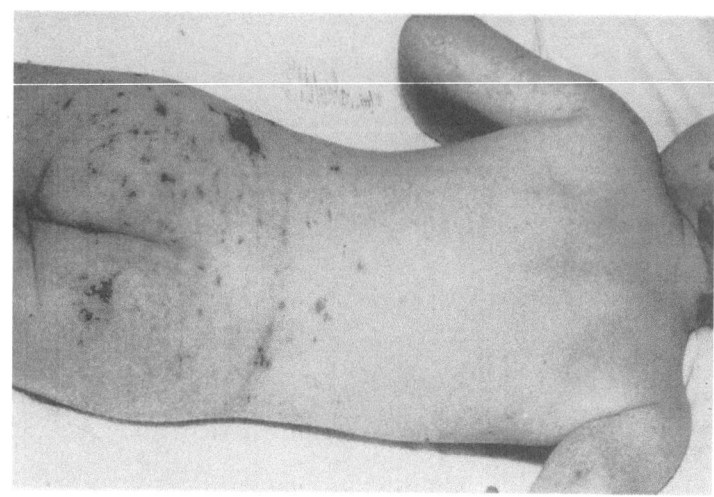

epidemics have occurred amongst adults in closed communities, such as barracks. Bacteraemia can occur in the absence of overt meningitis. Similar skin and joint lesions are found in pneumococcal bacteraemia.

8.1.4   Infective endocarditis

This may be caused by several bacteria including alpha-haemolytic streptococcus. Features include polyarthralgia and skin lesions including splinter haemorrhages (Figs 8.4 and 8.5), Janeway lesions (red macules typically

Fig. 8.4 Splinter haemorrhages in a patient with infective endocarditis. Note also the small digital infarcts. Similar changes are found in rheumatoid disease. Splinter haemorrhages are also seen in primary nail disorders such as psoriasis or fungal nail disease. Trauma is a very common cause of splinter haemorrhages.

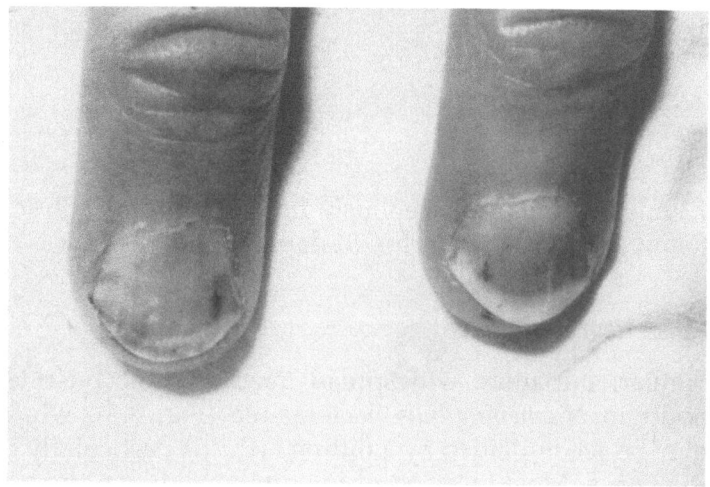

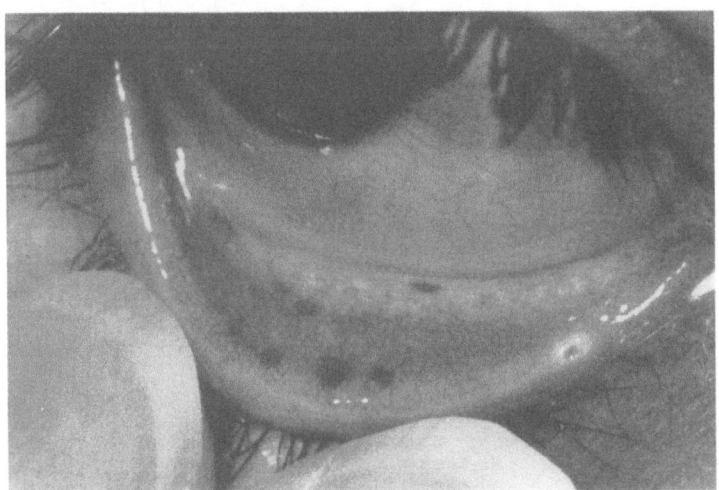

Fig. 8.5 Splinter haemorrhages on the conjunctivae in a patient with infective endocarditis. (Courtesy of Dr R. D. Thomas.)

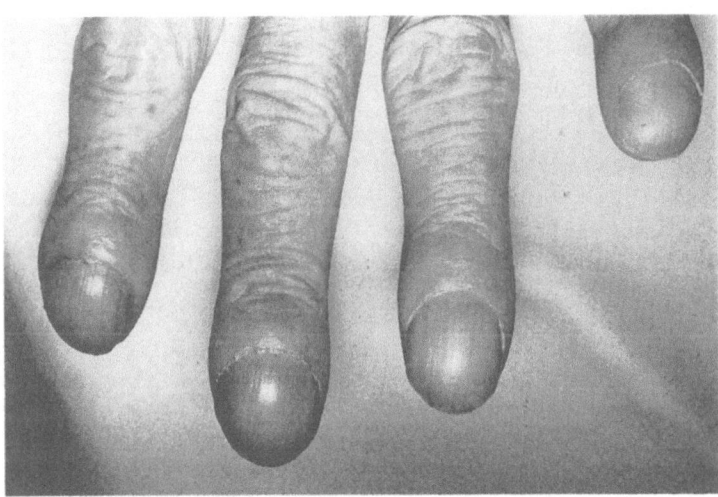

Fig. 8.6 Clubbing with obliteration of nail angle and increased curvature of the nail in a patient with infective endocarditis.

found on the thenar and hypothenar eminences), Osler's nodes (tender papules on the tips of fingers and toes) and clubbing (Fig. 8.6).

8.1.5 Spirochaetal infections

Lyme disease

Borellia burgdorferi infection follows tick bites, usually from the genus *Ixodes* (Fig. 8.7). Erythema chronicum migrans occurs at the site of the bite and is an expanding

Fig. 8.7 Tick (*Ixodes* sp.).

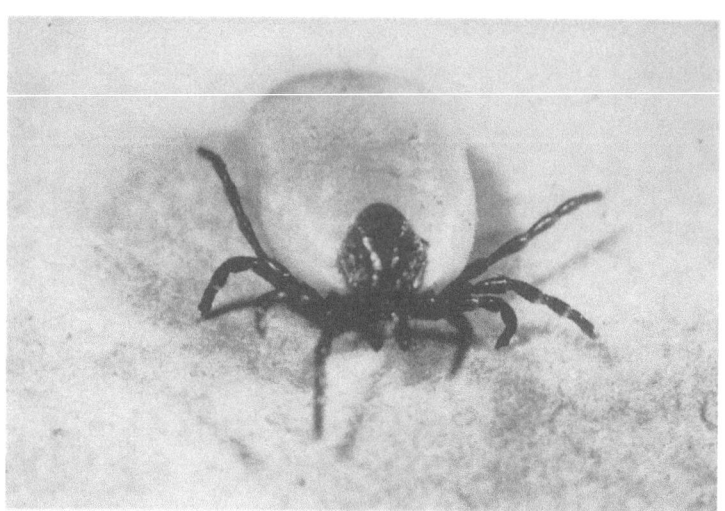

Fig. 8.8 Erythema chronicum
migrans. Expanding erythema
around site of tick bite.
(Courtesy of Dr E. Pascual.)

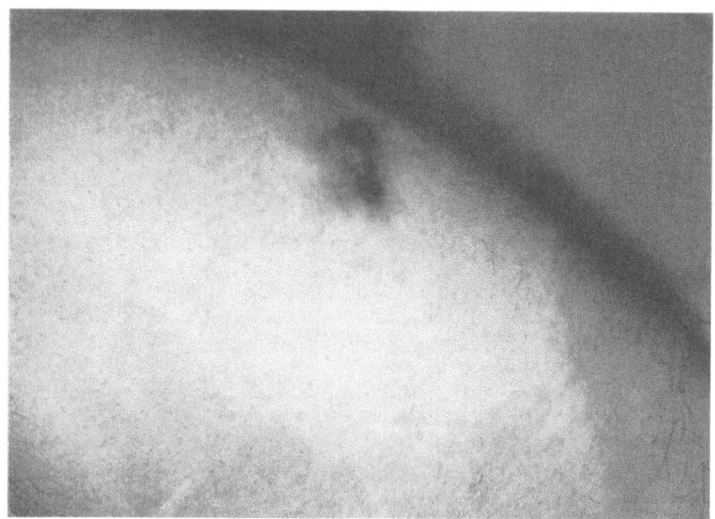

annular erythema (Fig. 8.8). In Britain skin lesions are
frequently the only manifestation but joint involvement, originally reported from Lyme, Connecticut, is
now seen worldwide. Joint symptoms are often abrupt
in onset and may be migratory, predominantly affecting
large joints, especially knees. Attacks typically last for
2 weeks but are recurrent and a chronic persistent synovitis may develop particularly in the knee. Systemic
features including cardiac conduction defects and neurological abnormalities may occur. The diagnosis can be

confirmed by detecting antibodies specific to *Borellia burgdorferi*. Antibiotic therapy with tetracycline may resolve early disease and prevent late complications such as persistent arthritis.

Treponema pallidum

In secondary syphilis a characteristic erythematous eruption involves trunk and limbs including palms

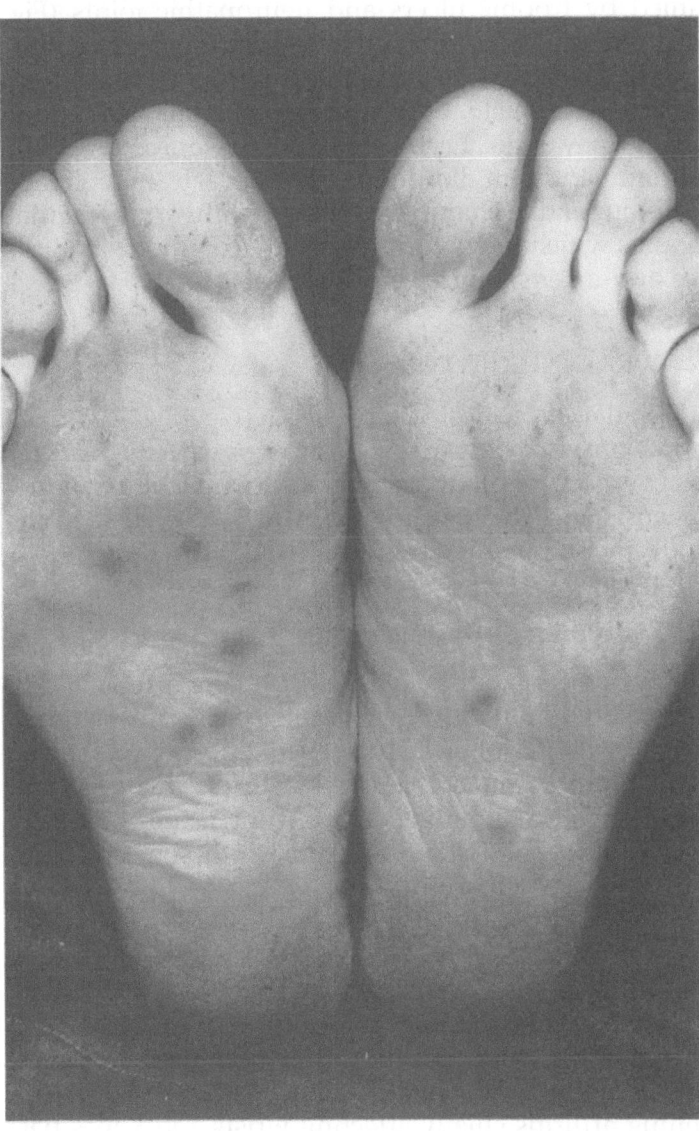

Fig. 8.9 Papules on the soles in secondary syphilis.

and soles (Fig. 8.9) associated with lymphadenopathy and sometimes arthralgia. Gummata, trophic ulcers and Charçot's (neuropathic) joints are features of tertiary syphilis. Saddle nose and Clutton's joints (swollen, cold knees) are features of congenital syphilis.

8.1.6 *Mycobacterium leprae*

Anaesthetic variably pigmented plaques and thickened nerves occur in tuberculoid leprosy, sometimes accompanied by trophic ulcers and neuropathic joints (Fig. 8.10). At the other end of the spectrum lepromatous leprosy is characterized by infiltrated cutaneous nodules teeming with bacilli. Local invasion of joints and tendon sheaths may occur. Erythema nodosum leprosum occurs predominantly in borderline leprosy. It may follow treatment and is characterized by painful erythematous nodules which may ulcerate and are commonest on the face and extensor surface of the limbs.

8.2 VIRAL INFECTIONS

A macular or urticated erythema (Fig. 8.11) and an abrupt onset of polyarthralgia are non-specific features of several viral illnesses including infectious mononucleosis and cytomegalovirus (CMV) as well as in the prodrome of hepatitis B infection.

8.2.1 Erythema infectiosum

This is caused by a parvovirus, B19. Characteristic skin lesions predominantly in children include a 'slapped cheek' erythema followed by a reticulate eruption starting on the buttocks and spreading distally (see Plate 5). Joint disease is more common in adult women and consists of a self-limiting peripheral arthritis. Both skin and joint lesions may be recurrent.

8.2.2 Rubella

A typical maculopapular rash starts on the face as well circumscribed pink macules, later becoming confluent and spreading to the limbs. It may be followed by a self-limiting arthritis chiefly affecting wrists and knees par-

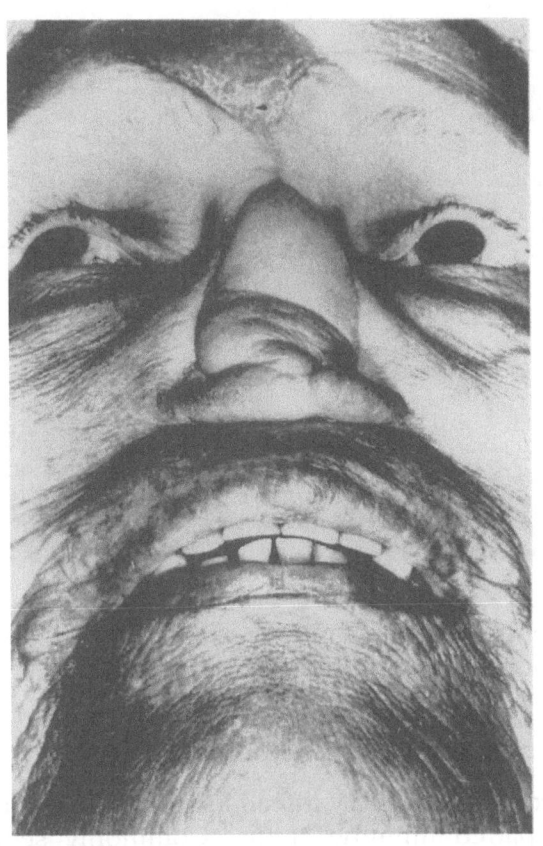

(a)

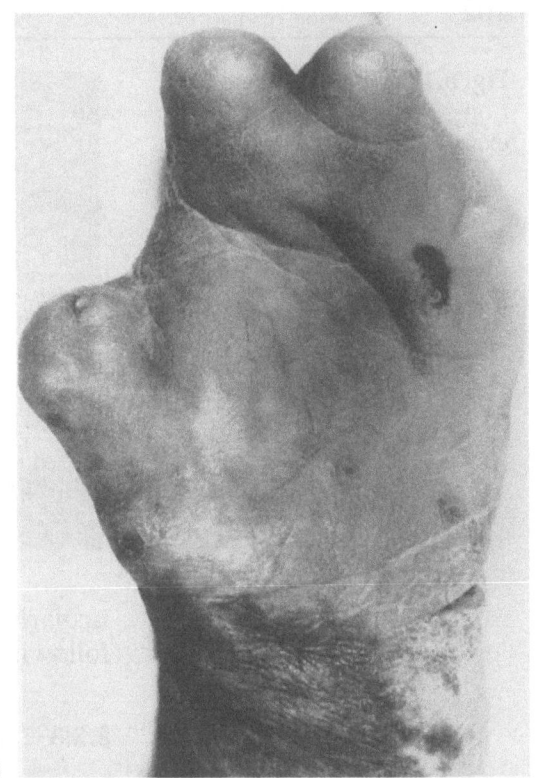

(b)

Fig. 8.10 Leprosy. Destructive changes affecting (a) nose, (b) hand and (c) foot. (Courtesy of Dr R. R. M. Harman.)

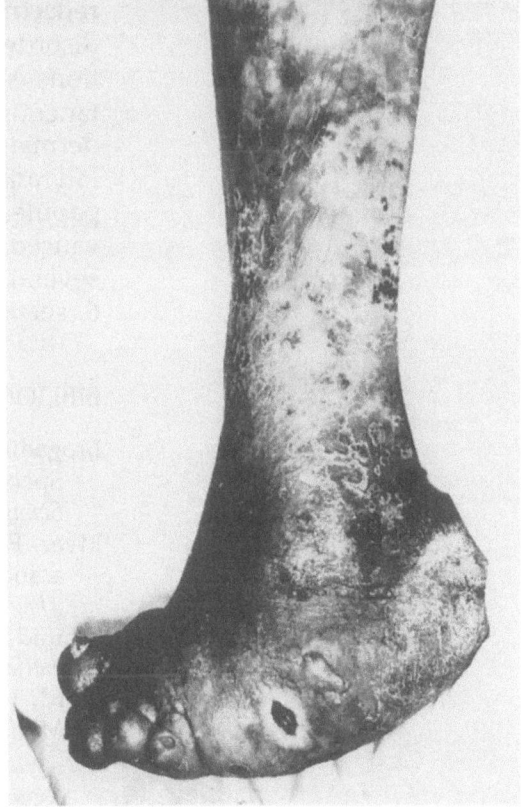

(c)

Fig. 8.11 Toxic erythema. A non-specific maculopapular exanthem.

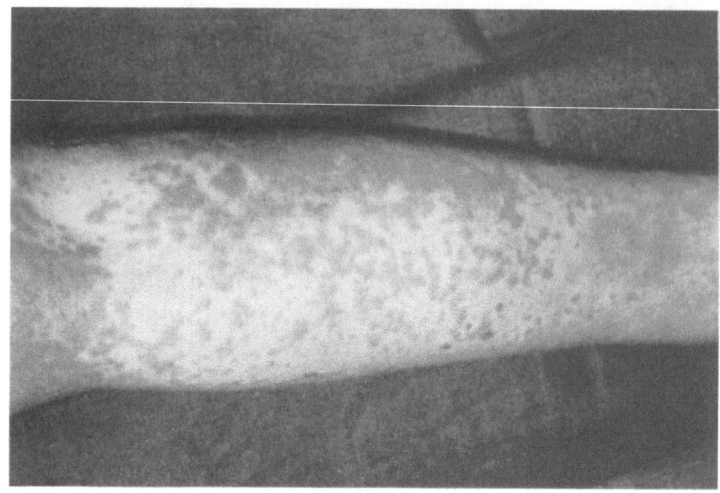

ticularly in young females. It may also occur a few weeks following inoculation with live attenuated virus.

8.2.3 Human immunodeficiency virus (HIV)

Many cutaneous signs of HIV infection are non-specific, reflecting impaired immune status. Commonly seen disorders may be exaggerated. These include infections such as herpes simplex, viral warts, mucocutaneous candidiasis, aphthae and florid seborrhoeic dermatitis (probably due to overgrowth of the yeast *Pityrosporum ovale*). The indolent bluish macules or papules of Kaposi's sarcoma are characteristic of advanced disease. Arthralgia is common and there are several reports of associated Reiter's disease (see Chapter 6, section 6.3).

BIBLIOGRAPHY

Brogadir, S. P., Schimmer, B. M. and Myers, P. R. (1979) Spectrum of the gonococcal arthritis-dermatitis syndrome. *Seminars in Arthritis and Rheumatism*, **8**, 177–83.

Myer, F. M. and Gottlieb, N. L. (1978) Rheumatic disorders associated with viral infection. *Seminars in Arthritis and Rheumatism*, **8**, 17–31.

Schmid, F. R. (ed.) (1978) Infectious arthritis. *Clinics in Rheumatic Diseases*, W. B. Saunders, London.

Ward, J. R. and Atcheson, S. G. (1977) Infectious arthritis. *Medical Clinics of North America*, **61**, 313–29.

CHAPTER NINE

Miscellaneous disorders affecting skin and joints

9.1 GENETIC DEFECTS OF CONNECTIVE TISSUE PROTEINS

Several syndromes have been described which incorporate hyperelasticity of skin with joint hypermobility. The commonest is *Marfan's syndrome*. Affected individuals are tall, with spindly digits (arachnodactyly). The skin may have an abnormal doughy texture and joint hypermobility is common. Cutaneous manifestations are more prominent in various forms of *Ehlers–Danlos syndrome* (EDS), the main forms of which are listed in Table 9.1. Cutaneous features include hyperextensible skin, skin fragility and bruising, 'cigarette paper' scarring, striae and molluscoid pseudotumours (Fig. 9.1). In type IV EDS distended blood vessels are apparent on the chest wall, associated with acrogeria and a high incidence of rupture of great vessels and bowel. Joint hypermobility is marked and is the principal feature of EDS type III. Hypermobility is complicated by recurrent dislocations and subsequent osteoarthritis. Thin skin and joint laxity are common features of *osteogenesis imperfecta*.

Cutaneous lesions in *pseudoxanthoma elasticum* (PXE) develop in early life as yellowish papules arranged in linear streaks in the axillae, sides of neck and groins (Fig. 9.2a and b). Joint hypermobility also occurs.

9.2 METABOLIC DISORDERS

9.2.1 Diabetes

The term *cheiroarthropathy* describes contracture of the joints, mainly of the fingers (camptodactyly), together with waxy cutaneous sclerosis occurring in association with type I diabetes (Fig. 9.3). Periarthritis, particularly

Table 9.1 The Ehlers–Danlos syndrome

Type	Name	Inheritance	Prominent clinical features			Underlying defect
			Skin hyperextensibility	Joint hypermobility	Other	
1	Gravis	Autosomal dominant	+	+	Cigarette paper scars. Mitral valve prolapse. Blue sclerae	?Defect of collagen fibre size and aggregation
2	Mitis	Autosomal dominant	+	+	Similar to, but less severe than 1. Easy bruising	?
3	Benign hypermobile	Autosomal dominant		+	Early osteoarthritis; probably commonest form	?
4a	Ecchymotic (acrogeria)	Autosomal recessive		±	Skin thin and pale. Easy bruising. Rupture of great vessels and bowel	Deficient type III collagen
b		Autosomal dominant			Similar to (a), but milder	
5	Sex-linked	Sex-linked recessive	+		Cigarette paper scars. Easy bruising	Deficient lysyl oxidase
6	Ocular	Autosomal recessive		+	Eyes { Blue sclerae / Microcornea / Rupture of globe / Retinal detachment } Aortic rupture	Deficient collagen hydroxylation
7	Arthrogryphosis multiplex	Autosomal recessive		+	Floppy baby. Short stature. Easy bruising	Structural mutation of collagen
8	Periodontitis	Autosomal dominant			Fragile skin Severe periodontitis	?
Other forms	e.g. Marfanoid, acquired cutis laxa	Autosomal recessive or sporadic	±	±	As above. Also Marfanoid habitus Increased skin laxity Platelet aggregation defects	Various, including deficiency of lysyl oxidase and fibronectin

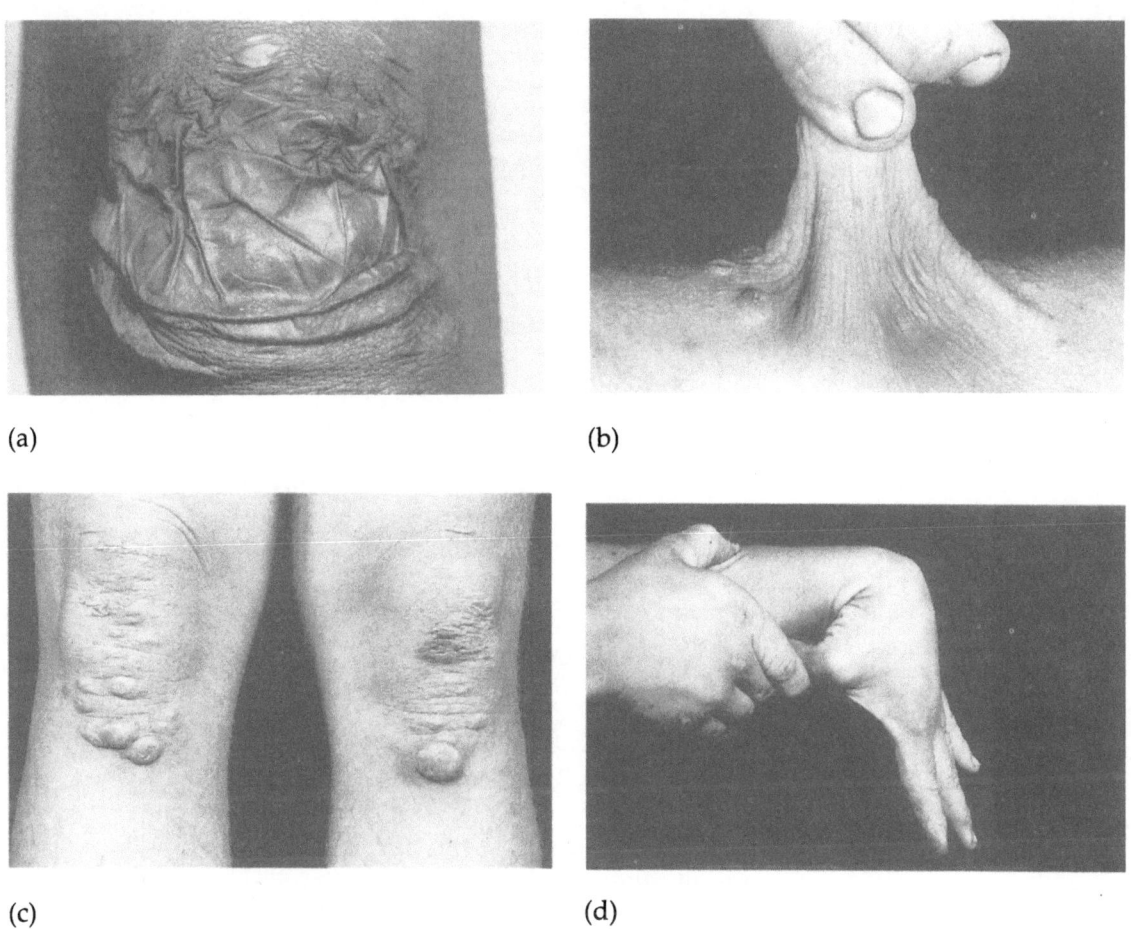

(a)

(b)

(c)

(d)

Fig. 9.1 Ehlers–Danlos syndrome. (a) Cigarette paper scarring on knee. (b) Hyperextensible skin and molluscoid pseudotumours. (c) Molluscoid pseudotumours and cigarette paper scars. (d) Hyperextensible joints.

rotator cuff inflammation, is also common in diabetics and there is an increased frequency of osteoarthritis. Trophic ulcers and Charçot joints are a late complication of diabetic neuropathy (Fig. 9.4).

9.2.2 Thyroid disease

Pruritus is common in both hyperthyroidism and hypothyroidism. Other cutaneous and musculoskeletal manifestations are rarer. Acropachy (Fig. 9.5) develops as a late feature in patients with Graves' disease. It presents with soft tissue swelling of the hands and feet and is

Fig. 9.2 Pseudoxanthoma
elasticum. 'Chicken breast'
papules on (a) neck, (b)
antecubital fossae.

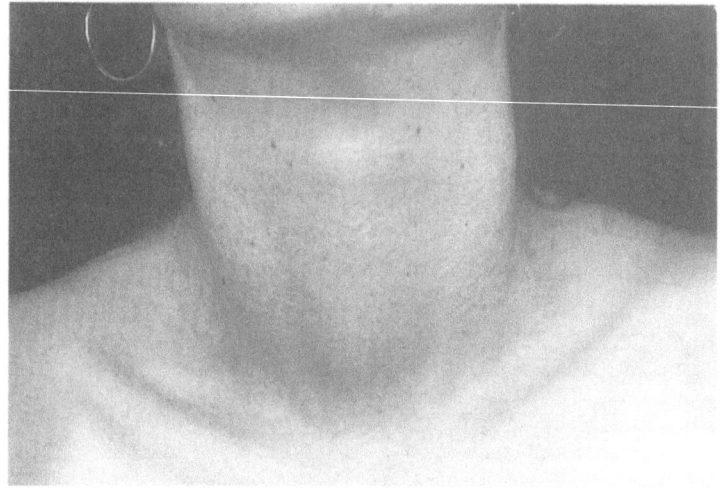

(a)

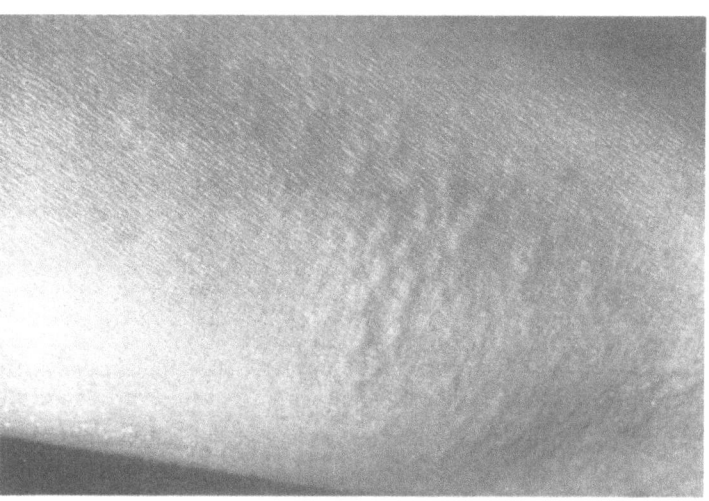

(b)

associated with clubbing and pretibial myxoedema (Fig.
9.6). Periosteal new bone formation is seen on x-rays of
distal long bones and phalanges. Florid myxoedema is
often associated with swelling and stiffness of peripheral
joints and large knee effusions, and responds rapidly to
thyroxine. Both hyperthyroidism and hypothyroidism
may be accompanied by a myopathy with weakness
predominantly of proximal muscles and marked eleva-

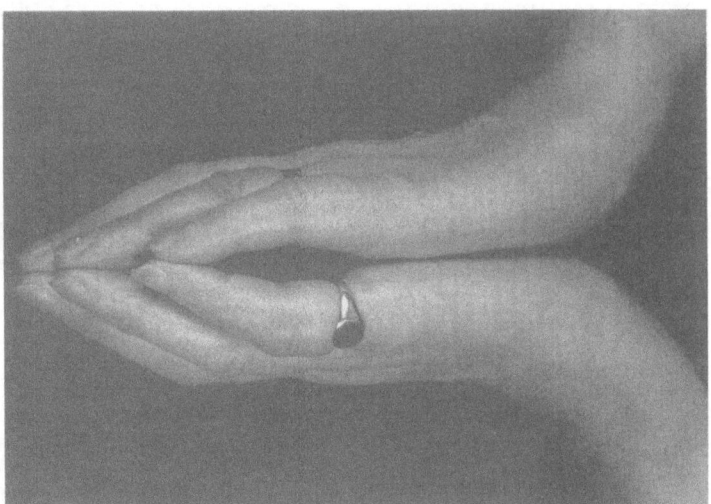

Fig. 9.3 Cheiroarthropathy in diabetes mellitus. (Courtesy of Prof P. A. Dieppe.)

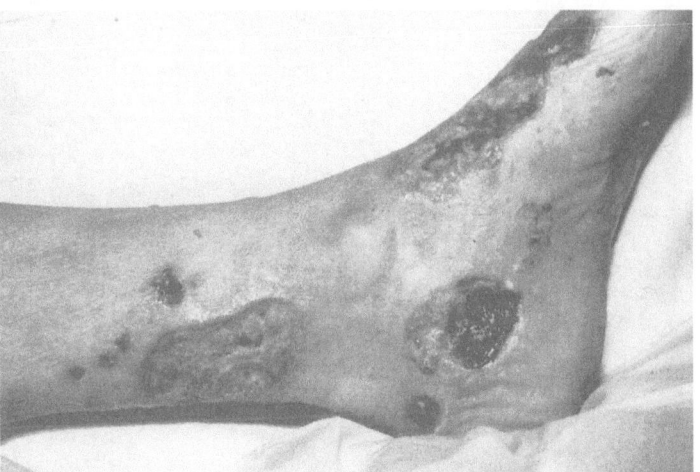

Fig. 9.4 Ischaemic ulcers in diabetes mellitus.

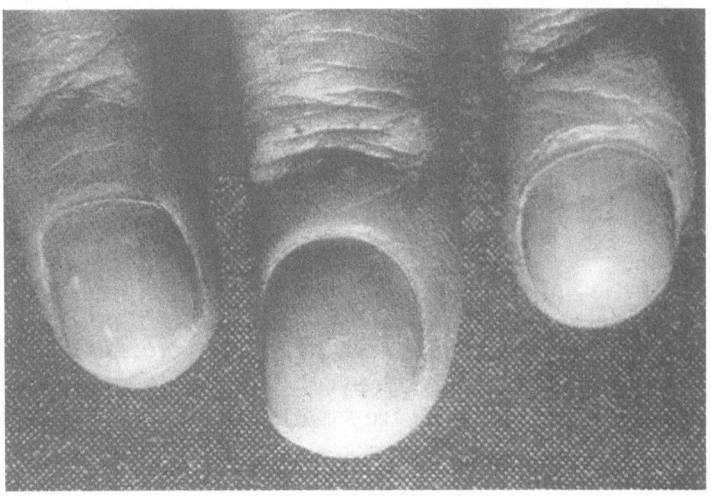

Fig. 9.5 Thyroid acropachy. (Courtesy of Dr J. Reckless.)

Fig. 9.6   Pretibial myxoedema.
Pinkish lesions develop on the
skin. Hair follicles may be
prominent. (Courtesy of Dr. J.
Reckless.)

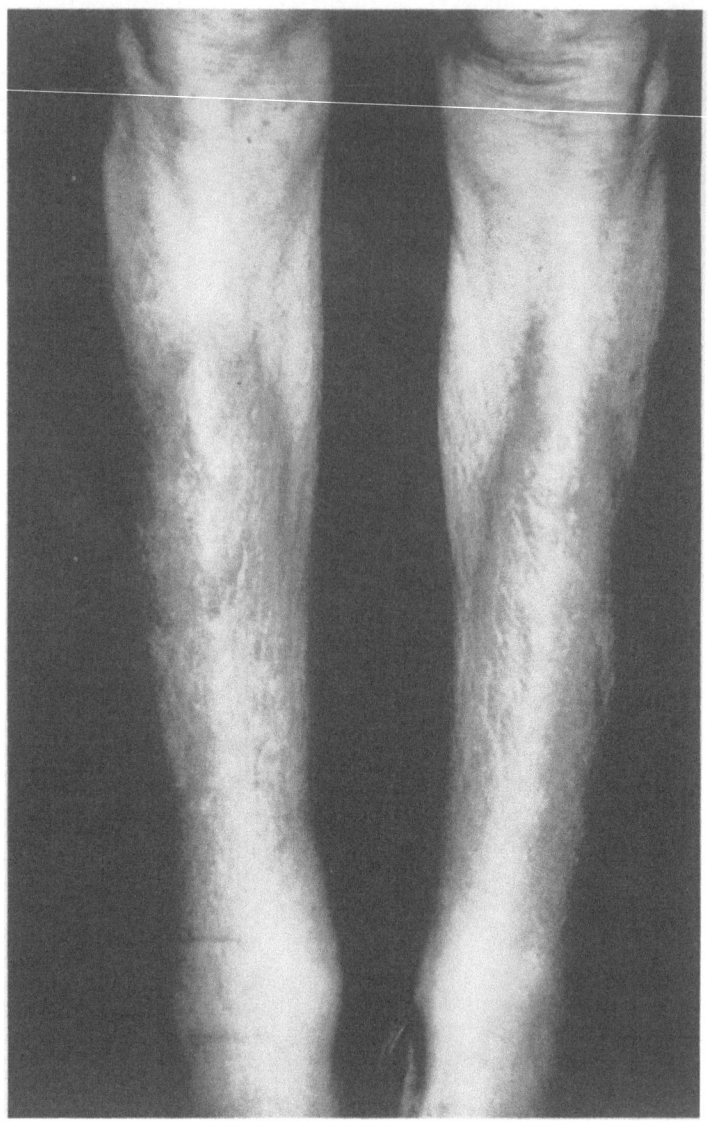

tion of serum levels of muscle enzymes such as creatine
phosphokinase.

9.2.3   Hyperlipidaemia

The association of skin and joint lesions occurs in familial
and in acquired hypertriglyceridaemia. In the former,
cutaneous xanthomata are associated with corneal arcus
and are florid in homozygotes, who develop premature

cardiovascular disease. A transient, migratory arthritis predominantly affects large joints. In hypertriglyceridaemia, eruptive xanthomata occur and joint symptoms may be non-specific. However, there is an increased incidence of gout.

9.2.4 Ochronosis

Deposition of homogentisic acid particularly in skin and cartilage results in blackening of the nares, pinnae, and sclerae (Fig. 9.7) slatey grey pigmentation, especially over extensor tendons and a progressive destructive osteoarthritis together with intervertebral disc disease. Homogentisic acid oxidase may be genetically deficient or related to drug ingestion. Similar changes occur in the skin following the use of bleaching creams containing hydroquinone (Fig. 9.8) and following antimalarial therapy.

9.2.5 Haemochromatosis

Increased tissue deposition of iron produces slatey grey skin pigmentation (see Plate 6) and hair loss. Premature osteoarthritis is associated with chondrocalcinosis. Deposition of iron occurs in many tissues including liver, heart and testes causing organ dysfunction. Diabetes mellitus is an important feature.

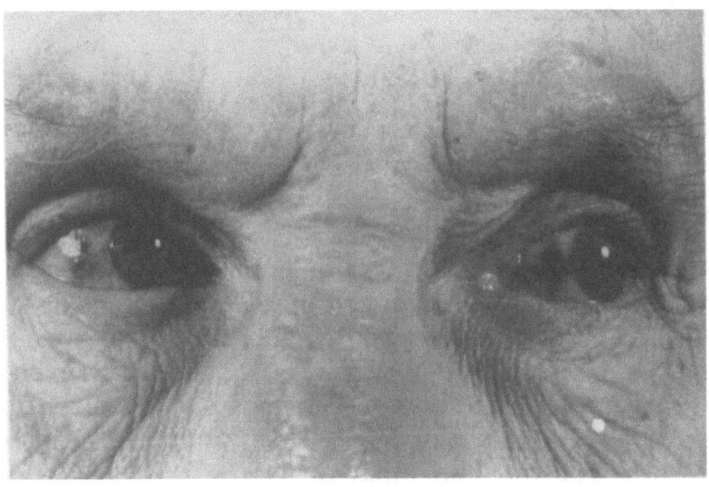

Fig. 9.7 Ochronosis. Scleral deposition of pigment typically occurs midway between the inner canthus and the corneal margin. (Courtesy of Prof P. A. Dieppe.)

Fig. 9.8 Cutaneous ochronosis due to the use of a bleaching cream containing hydroquinone.

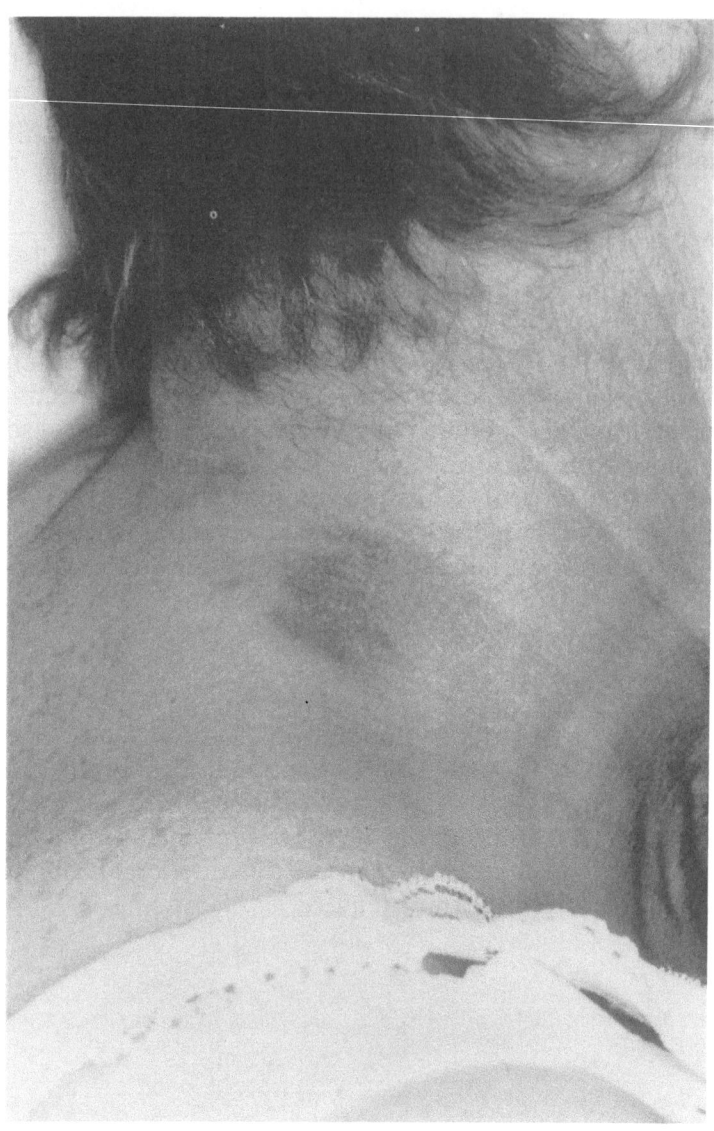

9.2.6   Scurvy

Ascorbic acid (vitamin C) is essential for synthesis of collagen and glycosaminoglycans. Deficiency leads to follicular hyperkeratoses on the limbs with areas of haemorrhage, initially perifollicular (Fig. 9.9) but eventually forming large areas of ecchymoses. Haemorrhagic effusions, especially of large joints, and painful subperiosteal haematomata may develop.

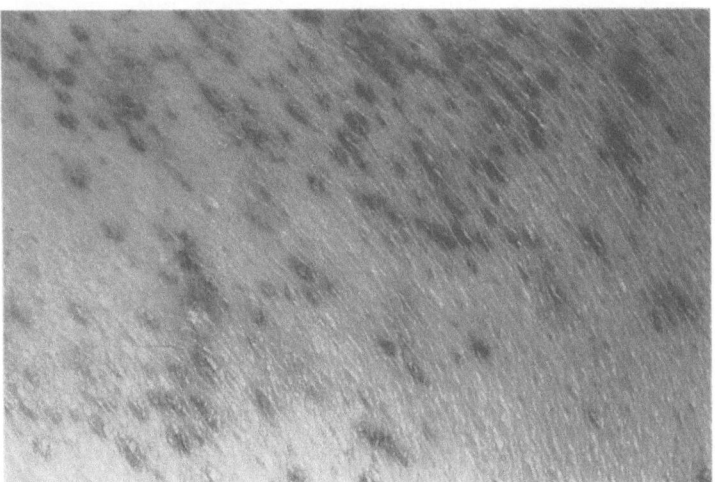

Fig. 9.9 Perifollicular haemorrhages in scurvy.

9.3 INFLAMMATORY DISORDERS

9.3.1 Still's disease

Typical onset occurs under the age of 5, both sexes being equally affected. Systemic features are prominent and include remittent fever, hepatosplenomegaly and serositis. A characteristic non-pruritic pinkish maculo-papular eruption occurs on the trunk and limbs (Fig. 9.10). The eruption is intermittent and often most marked in the evenings at the height of the fever. The wrists, ankles and knees are common sites of joint involvement together with the cervical spine. Up to 50% go on to develop chronic joint problems and amyloid may supervene in approximately 3%. A similar clinical picture may occur in adults, in whom the carpal joints are often affected and may fuse.

9.3.2 Sarcoidosis

This is a multisystem disorder typically characterized by the formation of non-caseating granulomata. An acute form presents predominantly in caucasian females with fever, malaise, lymphadenopathy characteristically affecting the hila (Fig. 9.11), erythema nodosum (see Chapter 6) and arthralgia. A frank synovitis may occur predominantly affecting the ankles and knees. Resolution is the rule.

Fig. 9.10 Still's disease. Numerous small macules with irregular margins. (Courtesy of Dr E. Pascual.)

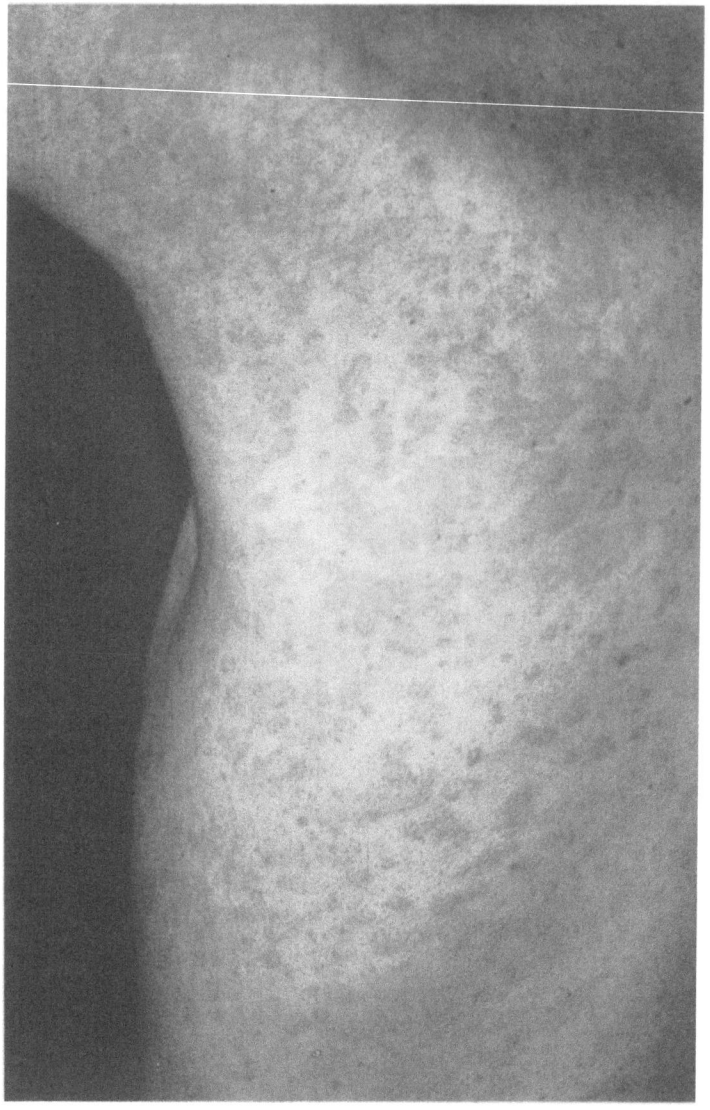

Chronic sarcoid is rarer and usually affects older patients. It is more severe in negroid races. Cutaneous and musculoskeletal involvement may be extensive and can occur in the absence of significant pulmonary involvement. Classical skin lesions are granulomatous (Fig. 9.12) bluish nodules, which may be hypopigmented in black skin with little epidermal involvement. They occur on the extremities, neck and back and sites of trauma (Fig. 9.13). Facial involvement is particularly

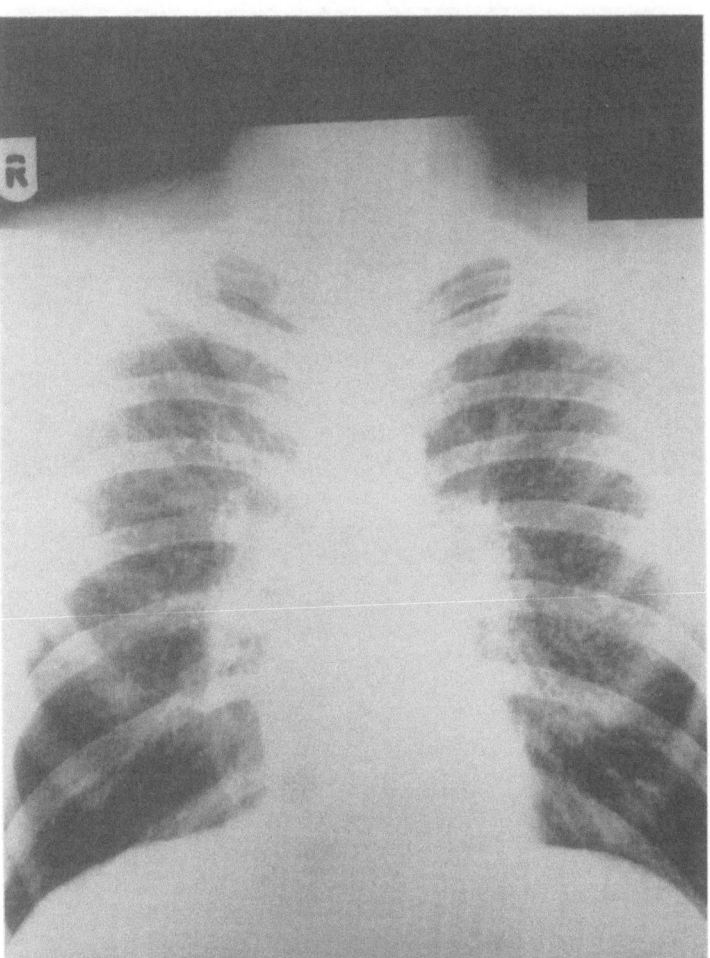

Fig. 9.11 Chest radiograph showing hilar and paratracheal lymphadenopathy with parenchymal infiltration. (Courtesy of Dr C. M. Higgs.)

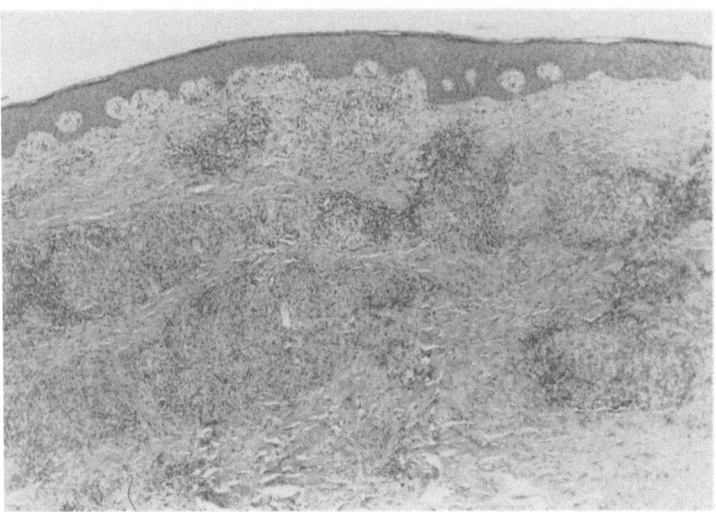

Fig. 9.12 Sarcoid granulomata in the dermis.

Fig. 9.13 Sarcoid nodules around the alae nasi in a West Indian patient.

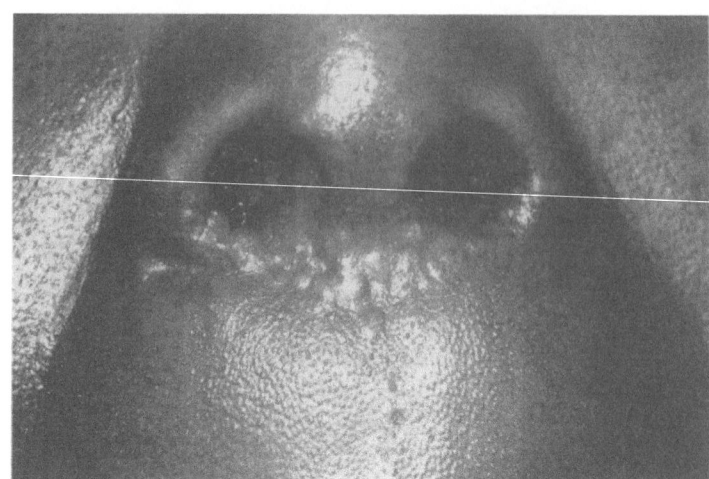

Fig. 9.14 Lupus pernio. A persistent bluish-red plaque or nodule, affecting principally the nose, occurs typically in middle-aged women with longstanding disease. Lesions may occur also on the cheeks, ears and fingers.

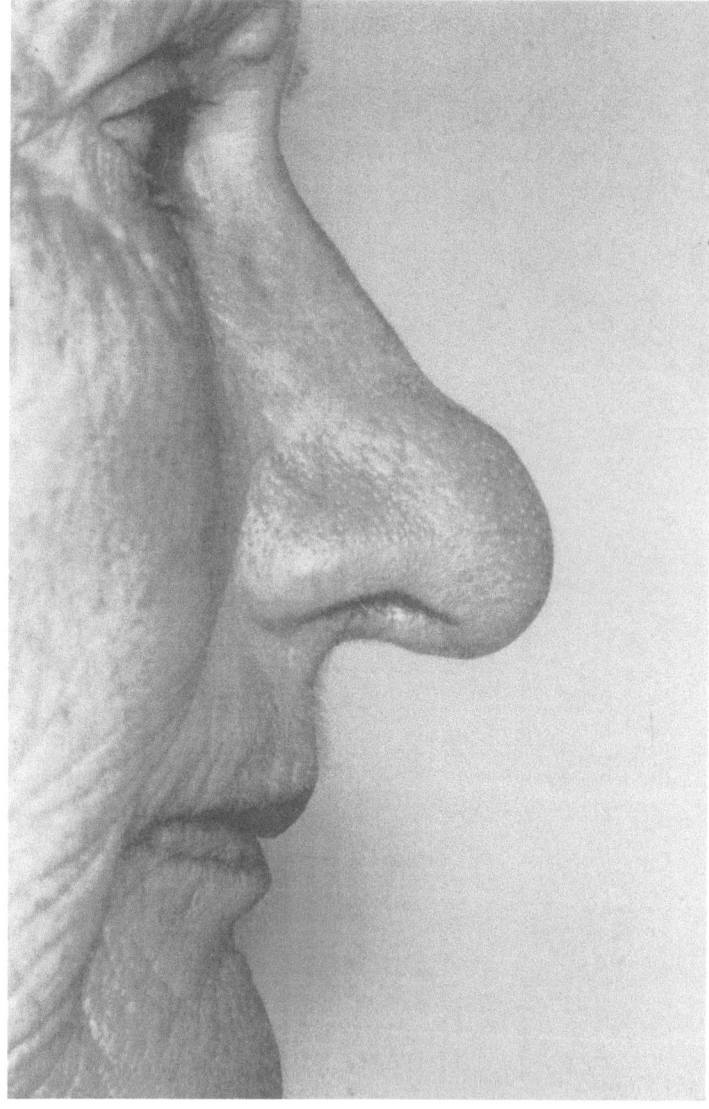

common in the negro. Diffuse infiltration of the nose is termed lupus pernio (Fig. 9.14). Prominent skin involvement is often accompanied by osseous lesions: these range from asymptomatic cystic lesions in the phalanges and metacarpals (Fig. 9.15) to florid dactylitis (Fig. 16a and b). Persistent arthralgia predominantly of knees, ankles and wrists can occur. Synovitis is rare in the caucasian. It may be episodic, resembling gout, or persistent in one or more joints; occasionally it may be symmetrical and resemble rheumatoid arthritis. It occurs principally in AfroCaribbeans.

9.3.3 Multicentric reticulohistiocytosis

This rare disorder predominantly affects the elderly and is often associated with internal neoplasia. The skin and

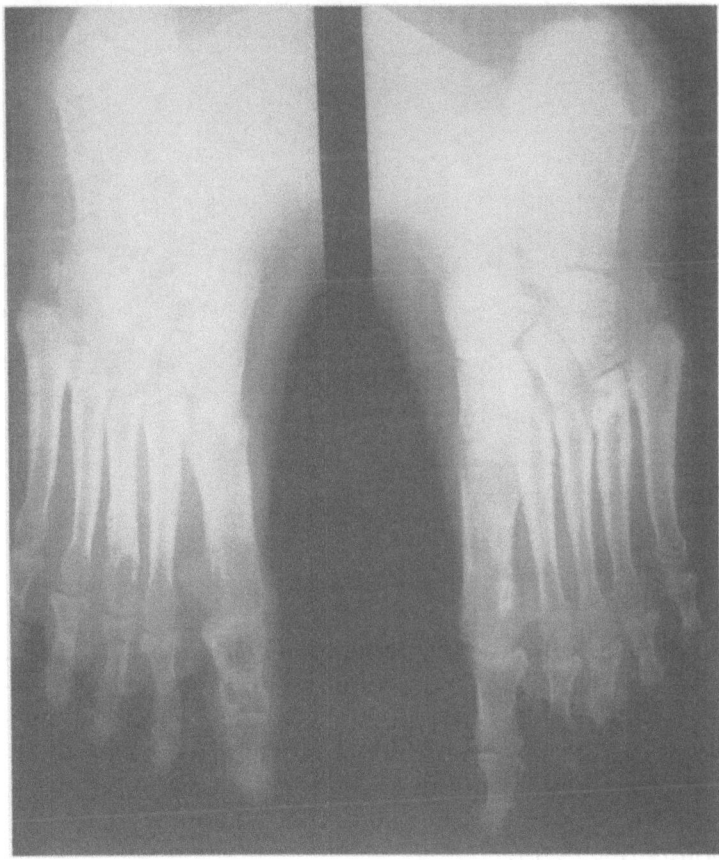

Fig. 9.15 Sarcoid dactylitis. Cystic lesions in phalanges.

Fig. 9.16 Sarcoid dactylitis.
(a) Numerous cystic lesions in
the phalanges, particularly
overlying joints. (b) X-ray of
hands showing punched out
cysts and "lattice-like" bone
lesions.

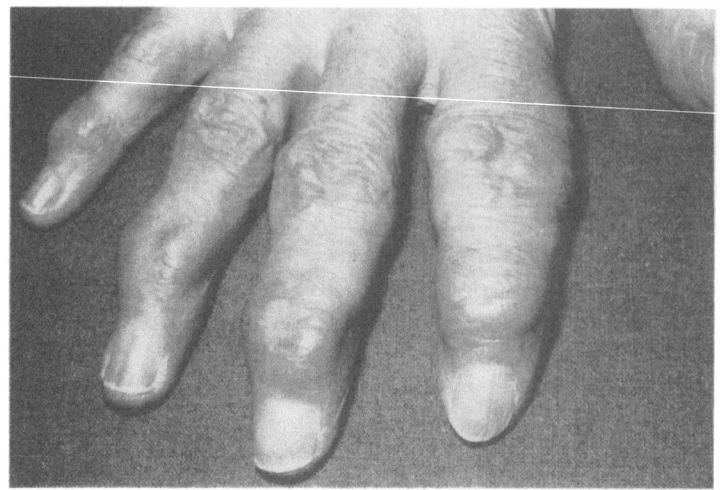

(a)

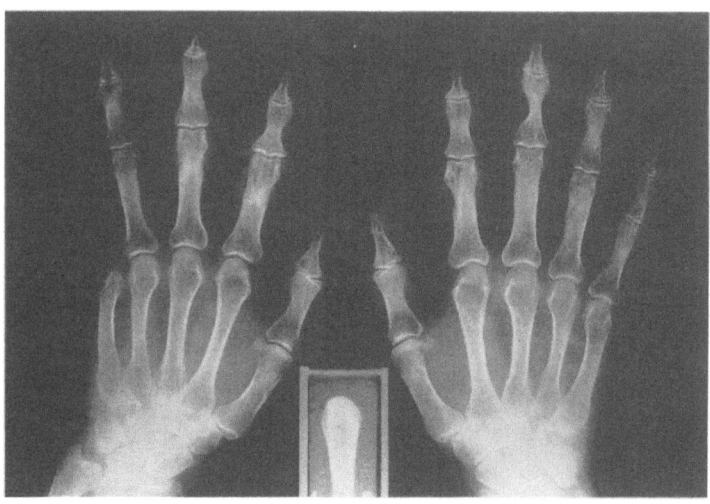

(b)

joints are infiltrated by foam-laden giant cells (Fig. 9.17).
Reddish-brown or skin-coloured nodules are characteristically found on the fingertips, around the nail
folds, nose, ears and trunk (Fig. 9.18a). Xanthelasmata
may develop around the eyelids (Fig. 9.18b). A severe,
erosive arthritis affects chiefly the distal interphalangeal
joints (Fig. 9.19).

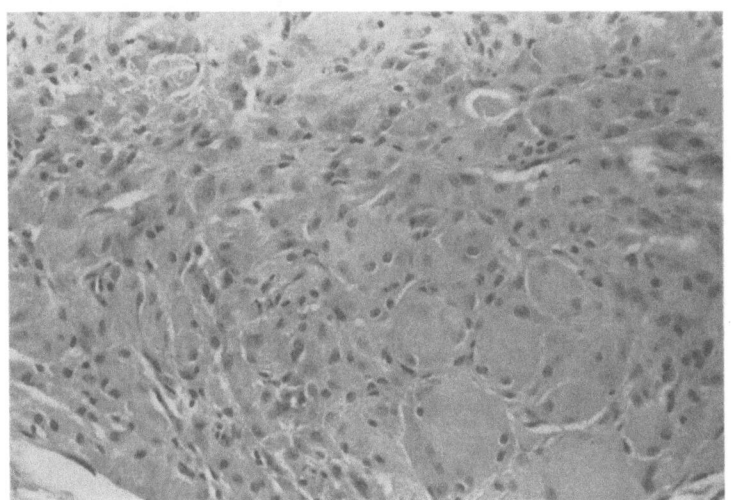

Fig. 9.17 Skin nodule in multicentric reticulohistio-cytosis showing large multi-nucleated giant cells with 'ground glass' cytoplasm.

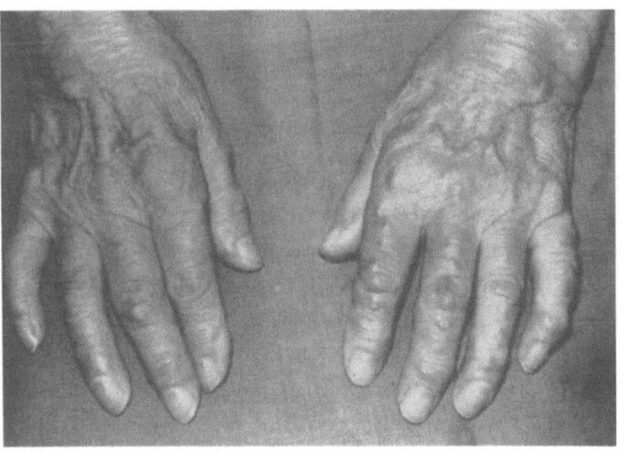

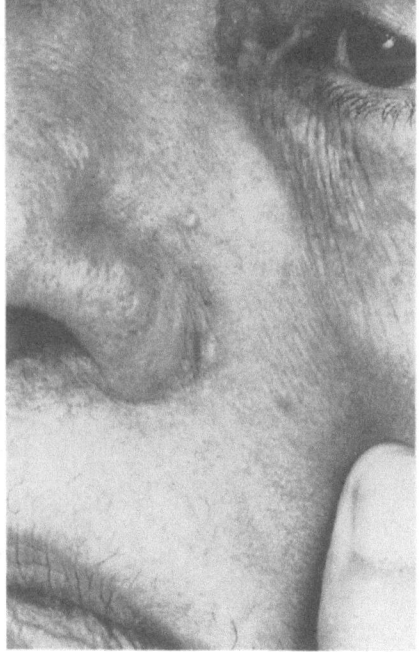

(a)   (b)

Fig. 9.18 Multicentric reticulohistiocytosis. (a) Numerous skin-coloured or brownish papules are found particularly over the extensor aspects of finger joints. (b) Xanthelasma palpebrarum and papules in nasolabial folds.

Fig. 9.19 Radiograph showing juxta-articular bone resorption in multicentric reticulo-histiocytosis.

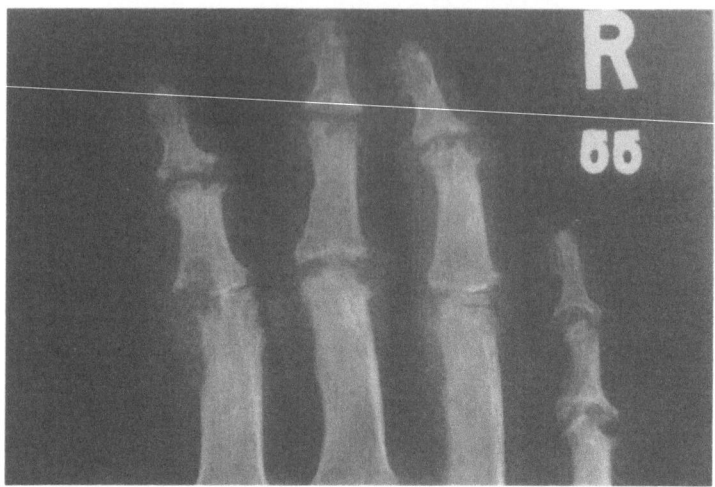

9.3.4   Sweet's syndrome (acute neutrophilic dermatosis)

This is a rare condition in which raised plum-coloured lesions (Plate 7) occur typically around the head and neck accompanied by fever, leucocytosis and often an acute arthritis of peripheral joints. Skin biopsy shows dense infiltration of neutrophils in the dermis (Fig. 9.20).

9.3.5   Behçet's syndrome

The classical triad comprises recurrent oral and genital ulceration and iritis (Fig. 9.21). It is commoner in males. Oral ulceration can be indistinguishable from common aphthae but is usually more indolent. Ulcers may be shallow or deep with a necrotic sloughing base. Skin lesions include follicular or perifollicular pustules, which may be acneiform. Systemic manifestations include bowel involvement, cerebral thrombophlebitis and a non-erosive synovitis typically affecting large joints. A form of the disease is common in certain parts of the world such as Asia Minor and Japan where systemic features are commoner and it is an important cause of blindness. A positive pathergy test is diagnostic but rare in Europeans.

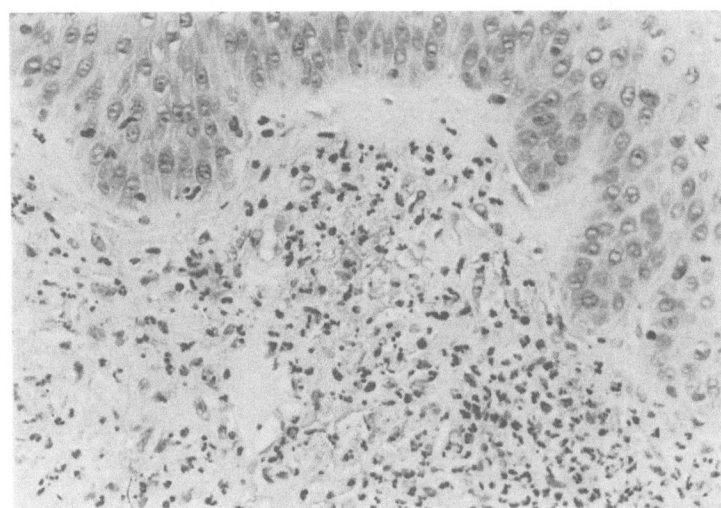

Fig. 9.20 Histology of Sweet's syndrome. A florid upper dermal infiltrate rich in neutrophils. (Courtesy of Dr T. I. Macleod.)

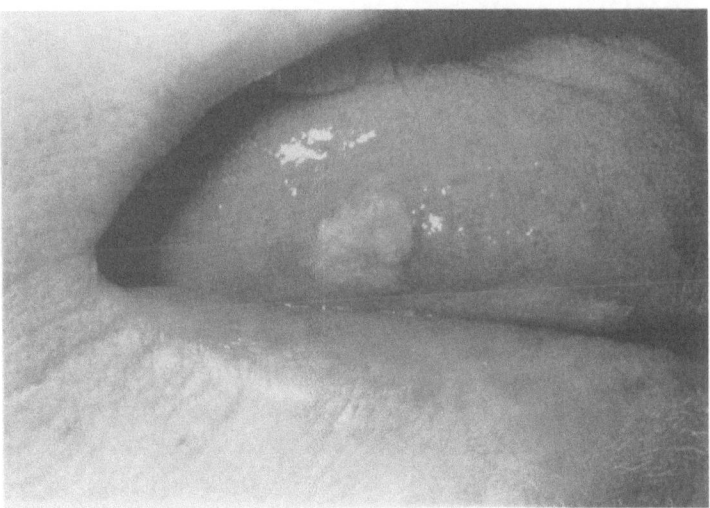

Fig. 9.21 Aphthosis in Behçet's syndrome.

9.3.6 Gout

Hyperuricaemia may be primary (often familial) or secondary (for example, from diuretic therapy). Self-limiting episodes of painful arthritis typically affect one, and later several joints. Later in the disease uric acid is deposited in cartilage (particularly the pinna), synovium and soft tissues (Fig. 9.22).

Fig. 9.22 Gouty tophi on the fingers.

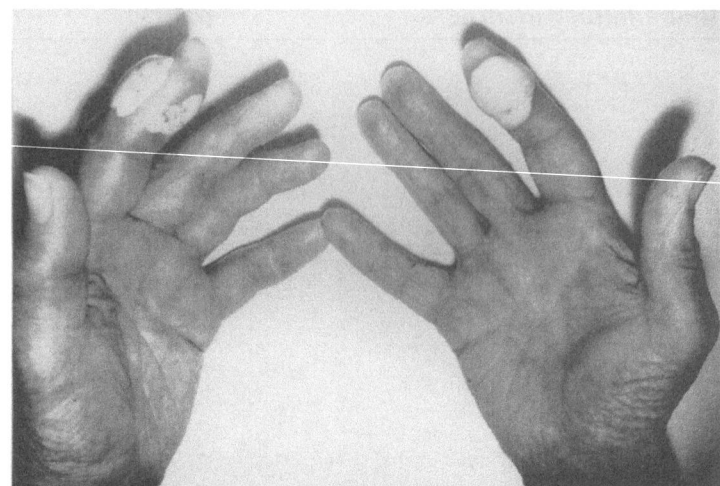

Fig. 9.23 Severe nodular cystic acne affecting the trunk.

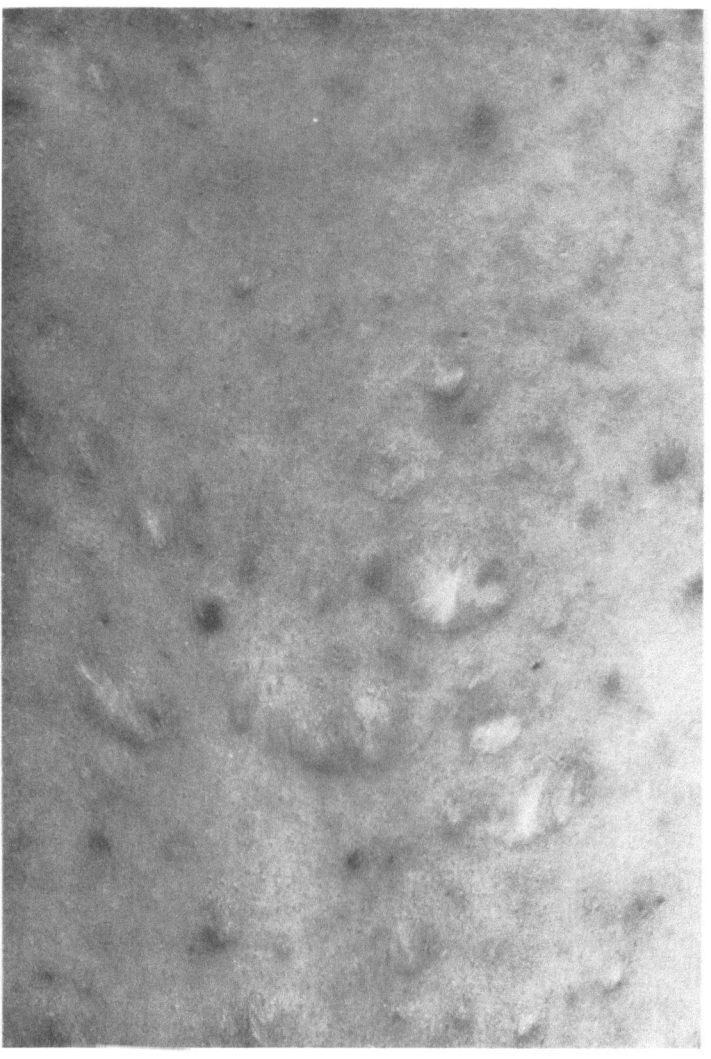

9.3.7 Acne fulminans

Rarely, males with severe inflammatory acne of the trunk develop fever, arthralgia and myalgia. Synovitis may affect one or several joints. Skin tests reveal extensive immediate or delayed hypersensitivity to propionobacterium acnes (Fig. 9.23).

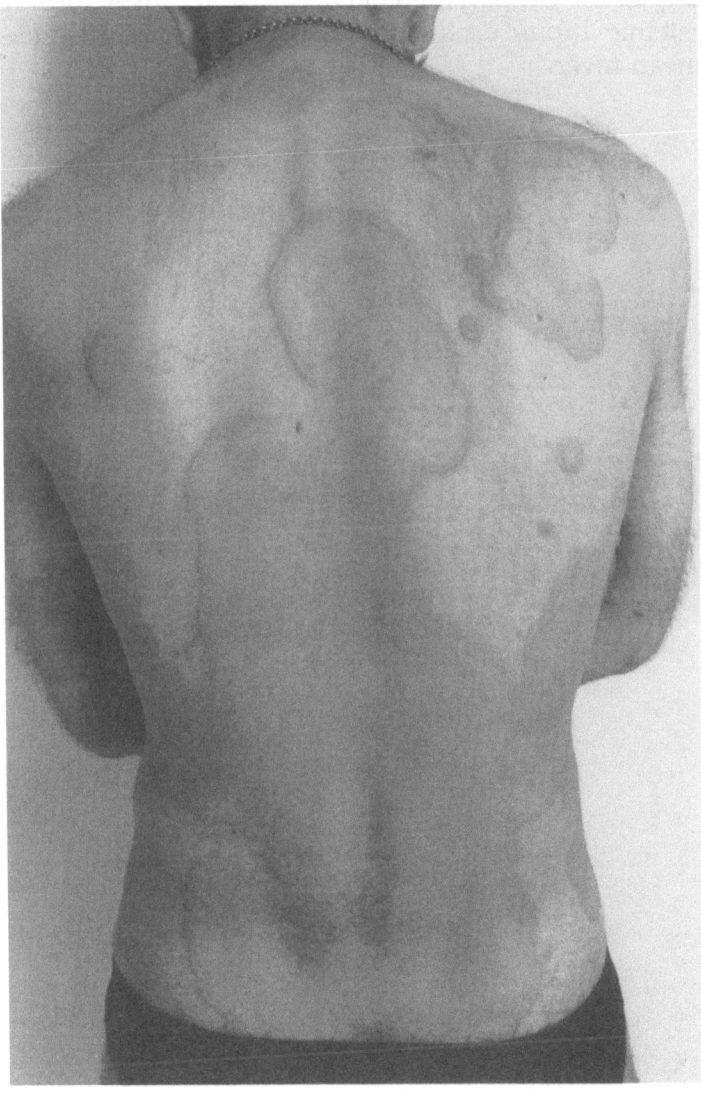

Fig. 9.24 Extensive urticarial plaques ('giant urticaria').

9.3.8 Urticaria

Transient erythematous papules, nodules or plaques are characteristically pruritic. Extensive cutaneous involvement may be associated with transient arthralgia. In simple urticaria an underlying cause is rarely found and the condition is self-limiting. Urticaria (Fig. 9.24) may be exacerbated by aspirin and related drugs. If individual weals persist more than 24 hours, are painful rather than pruritic, or resolve to leave bruise-like lesions, urticarial vasculitis should be considered (see Chapter 5). Underlying general medical causes include systemic lupus erythematosus and familial Mediterranean fever.

CHAPTER TEN

Cutaneous side-effects of antirheumatic therapy

Cutaneous drug reactions are frequent and a common reason for stopping therapy. Although frequently mild, on occasions they can be severe and even life-threatening – for example, toxic epidermal necrolysis. They may mimic a wide range of dermatoses from which they must be distinguished. The major types of reaction are summarized in Table 10.1

10.1 NON-STEROIDAL ANTI-INFLAMMATORY DRUGS (NSAIDS)

Cutaneous side-effects are usually minor, non-specific, maculopapular eruptions which may occur at any stage of therapy. Generalized exfoliative dermatitis occurs rarely and erythema multiforme has been reported with several NSAIDs. Photosensitivity is a rare complication of certain drugs in this class, notably fenbufen and benoxaprofen (now withdrawn). Skin fragility and onycholysis also occur. NSAIDs as a group and aspirin in particular can induce urticaria and even anaphylaxis via a pharmacological mechanism (see Chapter 9, section 9.3.8) (Fig. 10.1) particularly in patients with nasal polyposis.

Oxyphenbutazone, still used for ankylosing spondylitis, can cause a fixed drug eruption. As the term implies this is composed of one or more anatomically localized, sharply marginated erythematous plaques, sometimes bullous, resolving with scaling and dusky hyperpigmentation. The eruption recurs at the same site on re-exposure to the drug. Allergic contact dermatitis has been reported following topical administration of various NSAIDs.

Table 10.1 Important cutaneous reactions to antirheumatic drugs

Drug reaction	Non-steroidal anti-inflammatory (NSAIDs)	D-Penicillamine	Gold	Corticosteroids	Cytotoxics and immunosuppressives	Sulphasalazine	Antimalarials	Allopurinol
Maculopapular/exanthematic	+ (especially fenbufen)	+ (early)	+		± (especially azathioprine)	+	±	+
Erythroderma/exfoliation	+		+				+ (aggravate psoriasis)	+
Eczematous		?± (late)	+ (may resemble pityriasis rosea)					
Lichenoid		+	+				+	
Bullous: Pemphigus		+ (may mimic eczema)						
Pemphigoid Erythema multiforme and toxic epidermal necrolysis	+	+	±			+	+	+
Urticarial	+							
Fixed drug eruption	+ (especially oxyphenbutazone)							
Purpura	±	+	+	+	+	+	+	+
LE Syndrome		+						
Hyperpigmentation			+		+		+	
Photosensitivity and photo-onycholysis	+ (especially fenbufen and benoxaprofen)						+	±
Skin infections				+ e.g. folliculitis, candidiasis	+ e.g. viral warts			
Pruritus	+	+	+		±	+		+

+ = frequent
± = rare or doubtful

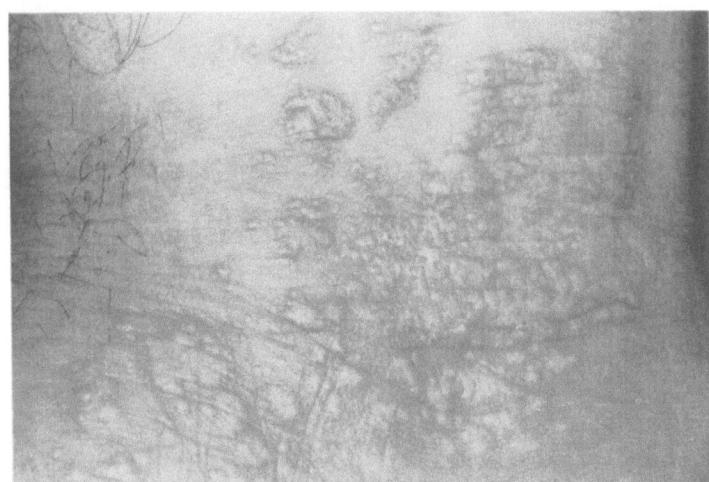

(a)

Fig. 10.1 Lichen planus due to penicillamine. (a) Polygonal papules with 'Wickham's striae' on the flexor aspect of the wrist. (b) Lace-like changes affecting the buccal mucosa.

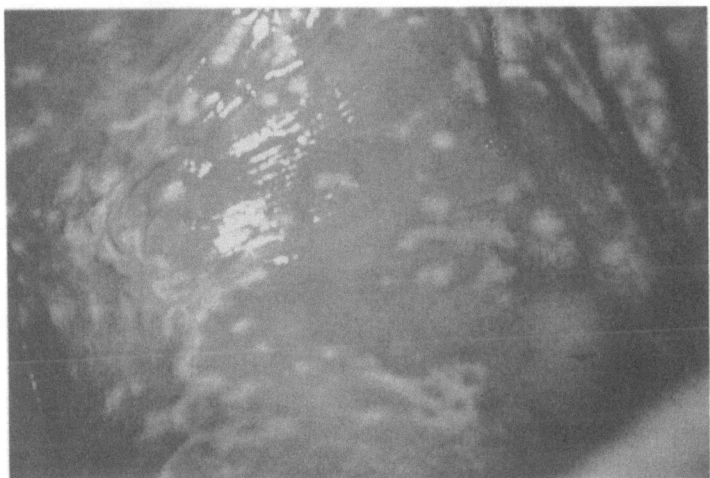

(b)

10.2 D-PENICILLAMINE

Skin manifestations are common particularly on higher doses (500 mg or more a day). The 'go low, go slow' regimen has reduced their frequency. Pruritus and maculopapular rashes occur early and can often be managed by temporary discontinuation and reintroduction on lower dosage. Late manifestations are more distinctive such as a lichenoid reaction which may be indistinguishable from lichen planus (Fig. 10.1) or a bullous eruption resembling pemphigoid clinically

Fig. 10.2 Pemphigoid. Tense bullae on limbs may occur on clinically normal skin or be surrounded by erythema and induration.

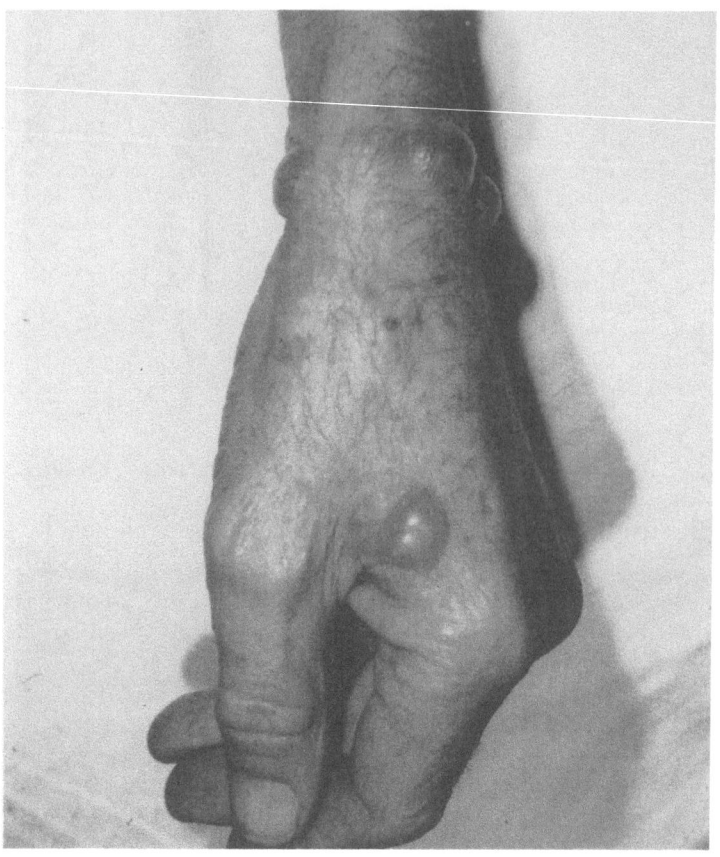

and histologically (Fig. 10.2). Cicatricial pemphigoid, affecting mucous membranes, is a rare manifestation, leading to oesophageal strictures and visual impairment due to conjunctival fibrous adhesions (synechiae).

More characteristic is an eruption resembling pemphigus foliaceus. A mild example is shown in Fig. 10.3. The lesions are chiefly truncal, indurated and crusted and superficially may resemble discrete areas of eczema. Frankly bullous pemphigus (vulgaris) is rarer (Fig. 10.4). The diagnosis should be confirmed histologically and by direct or indirect immunofluorescence which reveals the characteristic intercellular deposits of immunoglobulin in the epidermis. Epidermolysis bullosa acquisita, which clinically resembles porphyria cutanea tarda, has also been reported due to penicillamine.

Penicillamine occasionally causes a lupus syndrome (see Chapter 3). Unlike other drug induced lupus, induced by hydralazine or procainamide, antibodies to

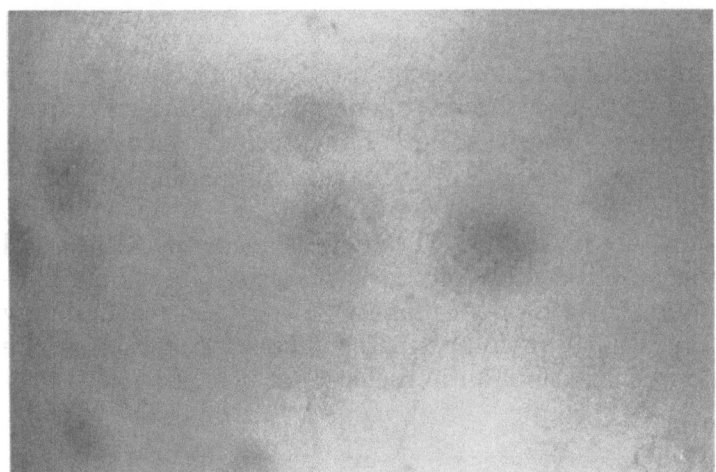

Fig. 10.3 Pemphigus foliaceus due to penicillamine. Superficial crusted lesions may mimic discoid eczema.

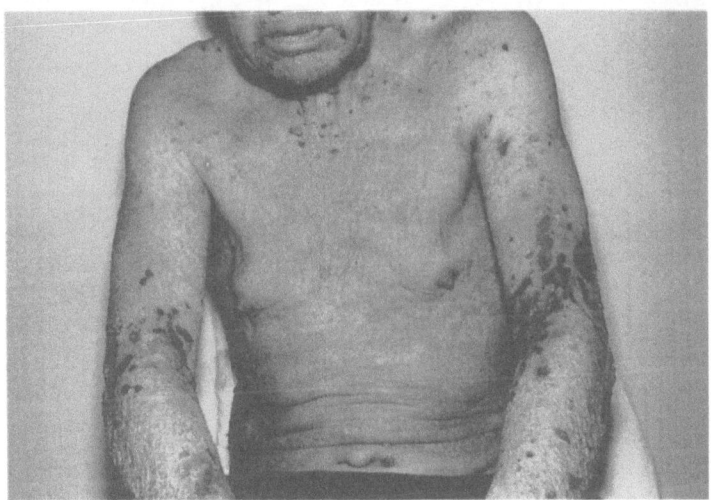

Fig. 10.4 Pemphigus vulgaris due to penicillamine.

native DNA are produced. Purpura is an important sign of severe thrombocytopenia due to bone marrow toxicity. Although minor cutaneous eruptions may respond to topical corticosteroids and temporary withdrawal of the drug, more serious manifestations usually require cessation of therapy.

Lathyrogenic effects on connective tissue (due to a direct effect on collagen cross-links) are rarely seen in the relatively low doses used in rheumatoid disease but elastosis perforans serpiginosa may occur. This presents as annular or linear groups of umbilicated papules, sometimes with a central horny plug, especially found around the neck.

10.3 GOLD

Cutaneous reactions occur in 15% on intramuscular gold at any stage of therapy, generally requiring its discontinuation. Pruritus and non-specific maculopapular eruptions (Fig. 10.5) are usually accompanied by eosinophilia. If the drug is continued they may progress to frank erythroderma. Eczematous reactions are typical and may resemble pityriasis rosea or seborrhoeic dermatitis. As with penicillamine, a lichenoid reaction may occur. Purpura indicates thrombocytopenia. Punctate stomatitis may occur in the absence of skin lesions. Pro-

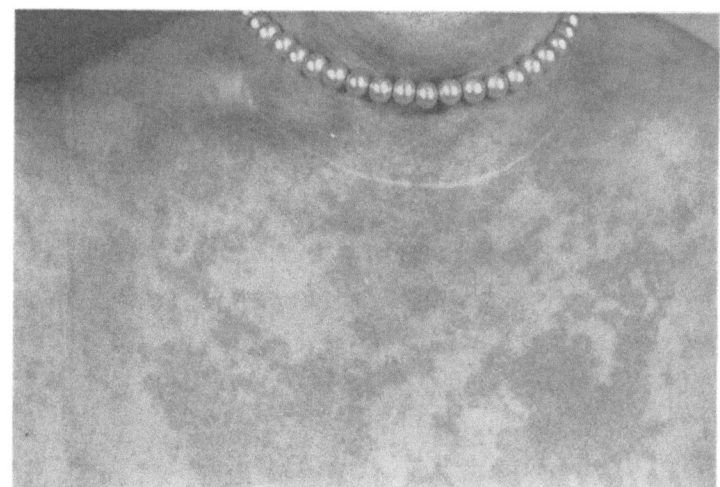

Fig. 10.5 Macular erythema due to intramuscular gold therapy.

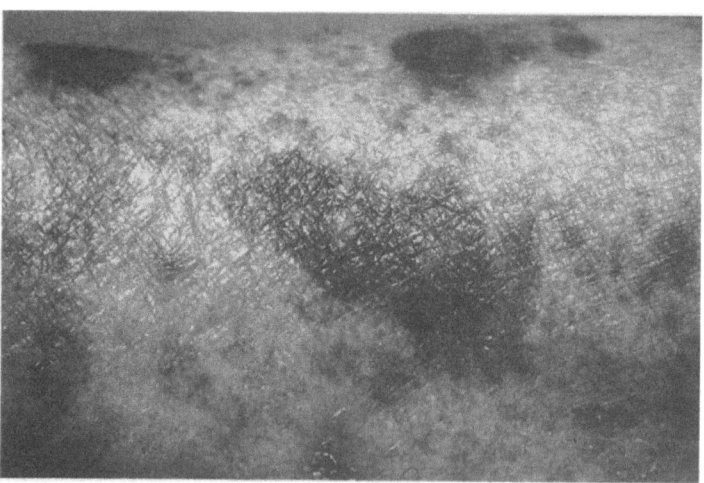

Fig. 10.6 Purpura and ecchymoses due to systemic corticosteroids.

longed chrysotherapy leads to diffuse slatey-grey pigmentation particularly of light-exposed skin. Experience
to date suggests that while the spectrum of cutaneous
reactions to oral gold is similar they are less severe.

10.4 CORTICOSTEROIDS

Prolonged corticosteroid therapy impairs collagen synthesis leading to skin thinning, fragility, striae, purpura
and ecchymoses (see Plate 8 and Fig. 10.6). There is an
increased tendency to cutaneous infection. Local injection therapy can lead to subcutaneous atrophy which
may be marked.

10.5 CYTOTOXICS

Cutaneous reactions are uncommon. Alkylating agents,
especially chlorambucil, are particularly liable to cause
bone marrow suppression which may present with
thrombocytopenic purpura. Immunosuppression pre-
disposes to bacterial and viral skin infections, particularly multiple viral warts and molluscum contagiosum.
There is an increased risk of cutaneous malignancy.
Stomatitis and orogenital ulceration are associated particularly with methotrexate therapy, while alopecia is
induced by cyclophosphamide. Exanthemata are rare
but are associated mostly with azathioprine. Pigmentation of the proximal nails has been reported in patients
taking cyclophosphamide.

10.6 SALAZOPYRIN (SULPHASALAZINE)

Reactions typically attributed to sulphonamides are also
seen with salazopyrin. They include maculopapular
eruptions, palpable purpura, erythema multiforme (Fig.
10.7) and even toxic epidermal necrolysis (Fig. 10.8).

10.7 ANTIMALARIALS

Like gold salts, antimalarials are deposited in the tissues
including the skin and the pigmented epithelium of the
eye. Diffuse greyish pigmentation occurs chiefly in light
exposed areas associated with increased melanin in
the basal layer of the epidermis. Diffuse yellowish

Fig. 10.7 Erythema multiforme due to sulphasalazine. Multiple 'target' lesions on the palms.

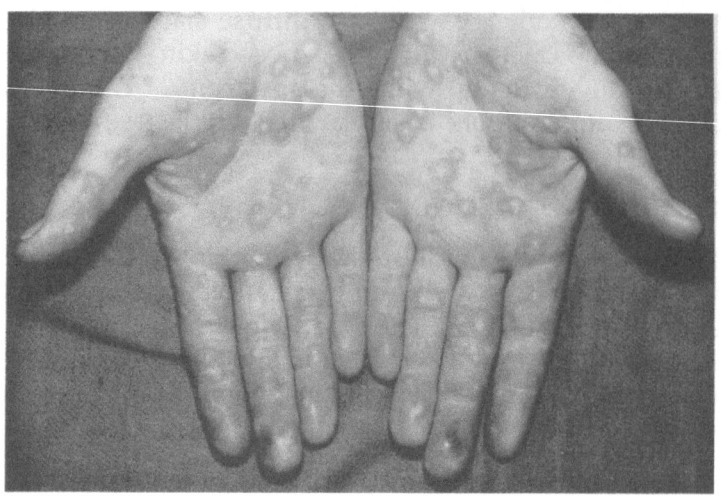

Fig. 10.8 Toxic epidermal necrolysis. Extensive shedding of skin leaving eroded areas. This may be a fatal complication of sulphonamide therapy.

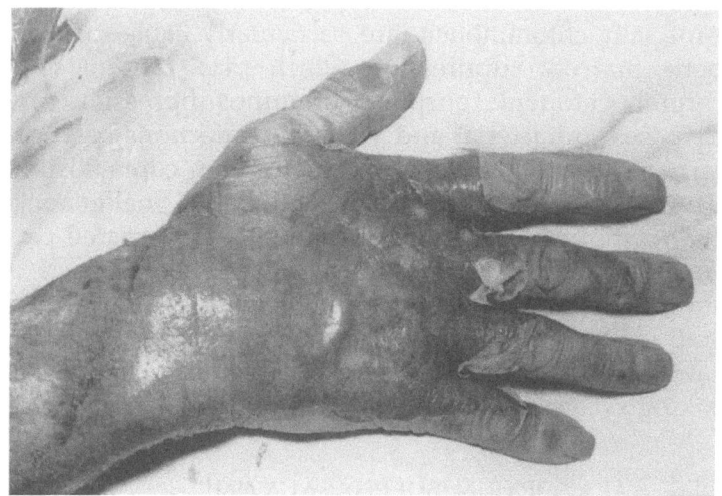

staining of the skin occurs in nearly everybody who takes mepacrine. It may also affect the conjunctivae and imitate jaundice. All antimalarials can cause acquired ochronosis. Conversely they can also bleach hair in blond and red-headed individuals. Drug-induced photosensitivity may occur and they can exacerbate cutaneous porphyria. Mepacrine in particular can cause a lichenoid eruption with a predilection for the palms and soles. Squamous cell carcinoma on the palms has been reported as a late sequel to this. Psoriasis can be exacerbated by antimalarials, sometimes severely.

10.8 ALLOPURINOL

This often causes pruritus, a maculopapular eruption and occasionally exfoliation. It is a cause of toxic epidermal necrolysis.

10.9 RADIATION AND OTHER PHYSICAL FORMS OF TREATMENT

Chronic effects of x-ray therapy, previously used for ankylosing spondylitis, include poikiloderma and multiple cutaneous carcinomata (Fig. 10.9). Repeated appli-

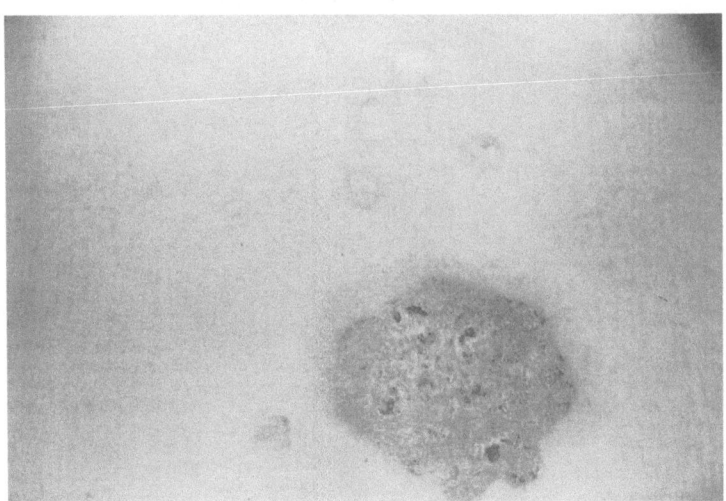

Fig. 10.9 Superficial basal cell carcinomata. Multiple lesions on lumbar region resulting from radiotherapy for ankylosing spondylitis.

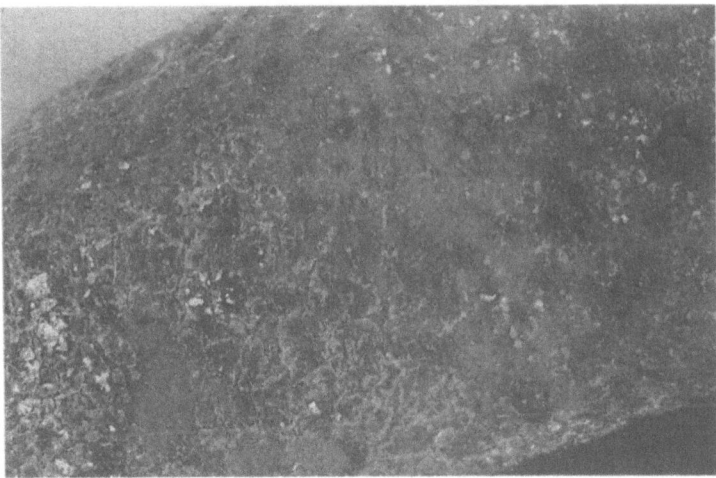

Fig. 10.10 Allergic contact dermatitis due to benzalkonium chloride, an agent added at one time to plaster of paris to prevent proliferation of *Clostridium tetani* spores. The acute vesicular eczema is localized to areas of contact with the plaster.

cation of hot packs to joints can cause erythema ab igne which must be distinguished from livedo reticularis (see Chapter 3). The use of plaster splints may induce irritant contact dermatitis and more rarely allergic contact dermatitis (Fig. 10.10).

Similarly, a non-specific eczematous eruption has been linked with delayed hypersensitivity to metals such as cobalt and chromium used in orthopaedic implants and may be associated with loosening of the implant. Investigation of such patients includes patch testing to metals, such as cobalt and chromium, used in the implant. Prophylactic patch testing with these metals is *not* of value in patients awaiting joint replacement.

CHAPTER ELEVEN

Common diagnostic problems

11.1 ONYCHOLYSIS

This is shown in Fig. 11.1. Increased separation of the free edge of the nail can be due to intrinsic abnormalities of the nail plate, producing abnormal nail growth or alteration of the nail bed, and/or extrinsic factors such as infection or trauma.

11.2 RAYNAUD'S PHENOMENON

This is episodic, multiphasic colour change associated with pain, paraesthesiae and numbness (Fig. 11.2 and Plates 9 and 10). Induced by temperature change, emotional stress or pressure. Classical sequence: vasospasm (white); stagnation of flow (blue); reactive painful hyperaemia (red). This sequence may vary. This may be due to:

(1) dysregulation of vascular smooth muscle tone, for example, idiopathic, beta-blocker induced
(2) intrinsic abnormalities of vessel wall, for example, connective tissue diseases
(3) increased viscosity, often cold induced, for example, cryoglobulinaemia
(4) entrapment syndromes, for example, thoracic inlet obstruction and carpal tunnel compression

Raynaud's is common in the normal female population (approximately 10%) and may be severe. A careful history should be taken to exclude exogenous factors such as beta-blocker therapy and the use of vibrating tools. 'Vibration white finger' follows the use of rotary or compressed-air tools such as pneumatic drills, chain saws and riveting guns. Symptoms may persist and even worsen after the use of these tools is discontinued.

Thoracic outlet syndrome should be considered in a young patient with asymmetrical Raynaud's. Clinical pointers to an occult connective tissue disease include

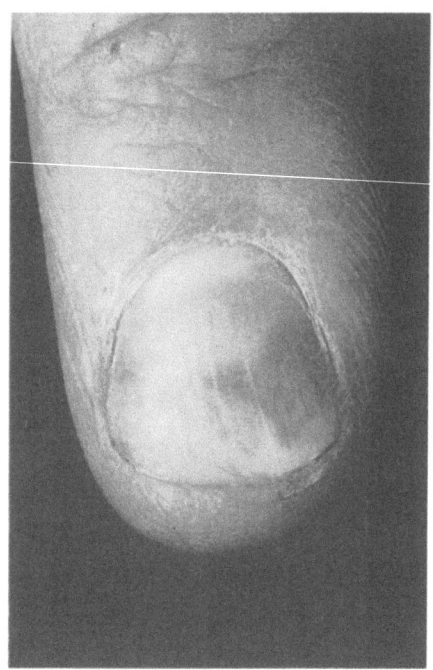

(a)

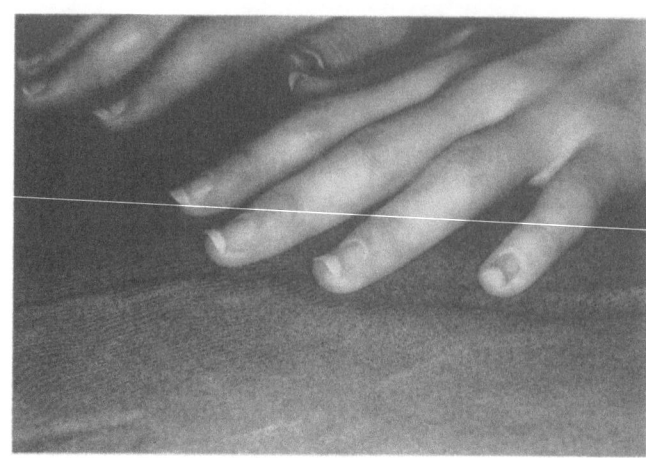

(b)

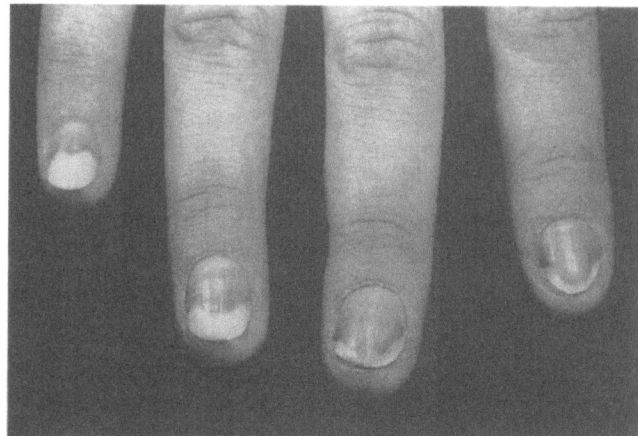

(c)

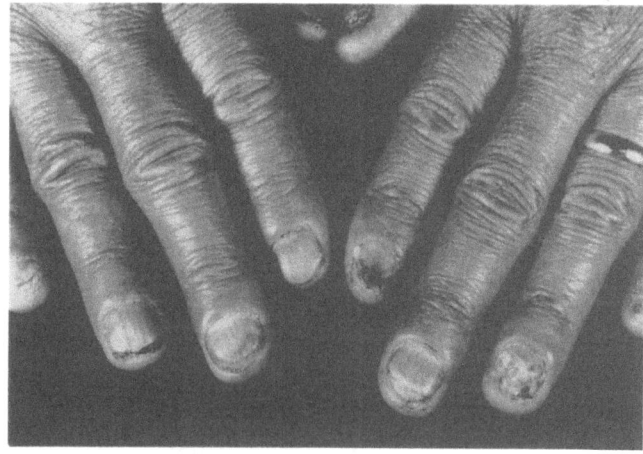

(d)

Fig. 11.1 Forms of onycholysis. (a) Psoriatic: irregular, often asymmetrical, associated with subungual hyperkeratosis, small deep pits, salmon patch and distal interphalangeal joint disease. Often intermittent affecting a variable number of nails. Similar abnormalities are seen in Reiter's disease.
(b) Connective tissue disease: uncommon, usually associated with Raynaud's. Symmetrical without hyperkeratosis but there may be ridging and associated nail fold abnormalities.
(c) Photo-onycholysis: usually drug-induced, especially tetracyclines and NSAIDs. Typically seasonal. (d) Fungal: often involves the whole nail matrix, particularly toe nails, typically asymmetrical with discoloration and gross thickening of the nail. Associated hyperkeratosis and maceration of the digital webs. Diagnosis can be made by microscopic examination of nail clippings and toe-web scrapings.

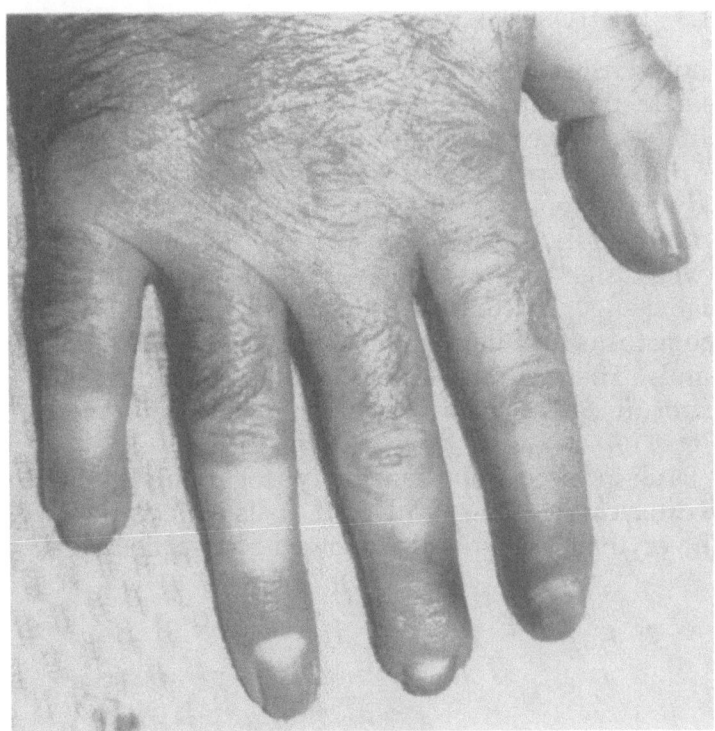

Fig. 11.2 Raynaud's phenomenon. Asymmetrical pallor of digits.

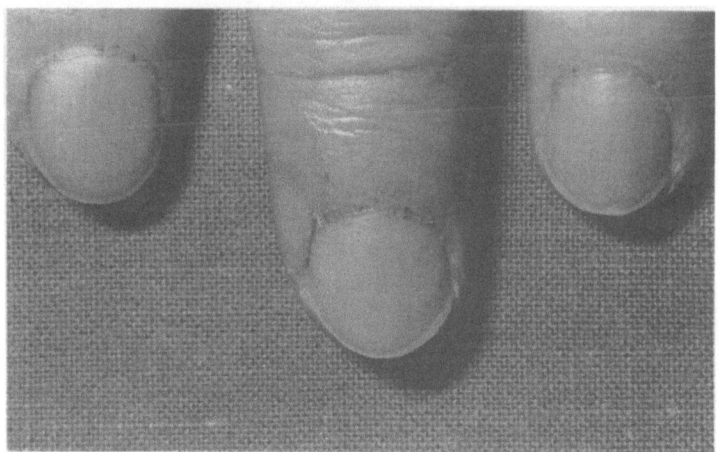

Fig. 11.3 Nail fold changes in a patient with Raynaud's secondary to lupus erythematosus.

digital ischaemic lesions, finger pulp scarring, swollen digits and nail fold capillary abnormalities which include dilated and distorted capillaries with areas of capillary loss (Fig. 11.3). Serological pointers include anticentromere antibody and other autoantibodies specific to connective tissue diseases.

11.3 PHOTOSENSITIVITY

Photosensitive eruptions are common in the normal female population and must be distinguished from photosensitivity secondary to connective tissue disease or drug therapy; 10% of women develop polymorphic light eruption, a pruritic papular eruption occurring within hours of sun exposure typically on normally covered sites and resolving within days without epidermal change. In contrast photosensitivity in lupus erythematosus and dermatomyositis also affects face and hands. There is often a longer latent period after sun exposure, it is usually less pruritic and persists longer (Fig. 11.4).

Drug-induced photosensitivity, for example, due to hydroxychloroquine and NSAIDs, also affects the face. The erythema is typically followed by desquamation.

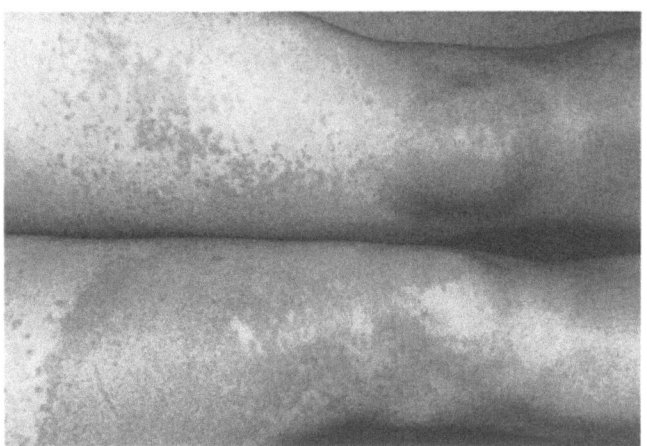
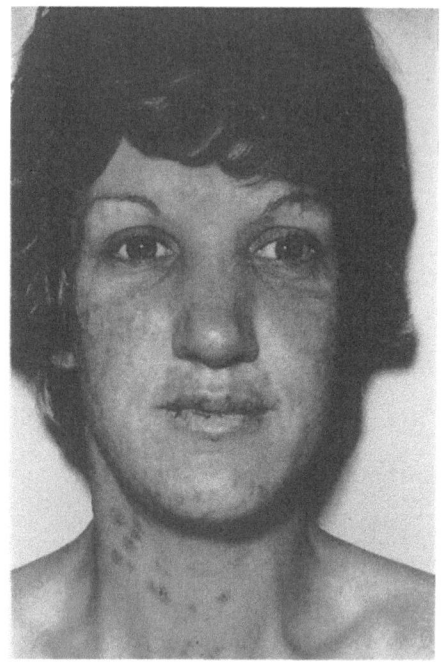

(a)   (b)

Fig. 11.4 Photosensitive eruptions. (a) Polymorphic light eruption. A papular erythema sparing covered sites (the patient was sunbathing wearing Bermuda shorts). (b) Involvement of light exposed areas of face and neck in SLE.

11.4 RED FACE AND SWOLLEN EYES

Facial erythema and periorbital oedema are typical features of dermatomyositis and systemic lupus and must be distinguished from non-rheumatological causes. Typical rosacea (Fig. 11.5) is papulopustular on a background of telangiectasia. A biopsy may be necessary to distinguish atypical forms. Benign lymphocytic infiltration such as Jessner's may produce papular or annular lesions indistinguishable from sub-acute and papular LE. Typical histological appearances include a dense dermal lymphocytic infiltrate without epidermal changes (Fig. 11.6). Seborrhoeic dermatitis may affect the cheeks and paranasal folds, is usually pruritic and associated with desquamation (Fig. 11.7).

The major differential diagnosis of eyelid swelling is allergic contact dermatitis in which eyelid swelling is acute in onset and resolves with scaling over a few days. It is often recurrent (Fig. 11.8). Eyelid swelling in angio-oedema is usually transient lasting a few hours. It resolves without scaling and is often associated with swelling of the lips or tongue. Other causes of bilateral eyelid swelling include nephrotic syndrome, hyper-thyroidism and hypothyroidism and superior vena canal obstruction. Erysipelas should be considered in a patient with acute unilateral eyelid swelling.

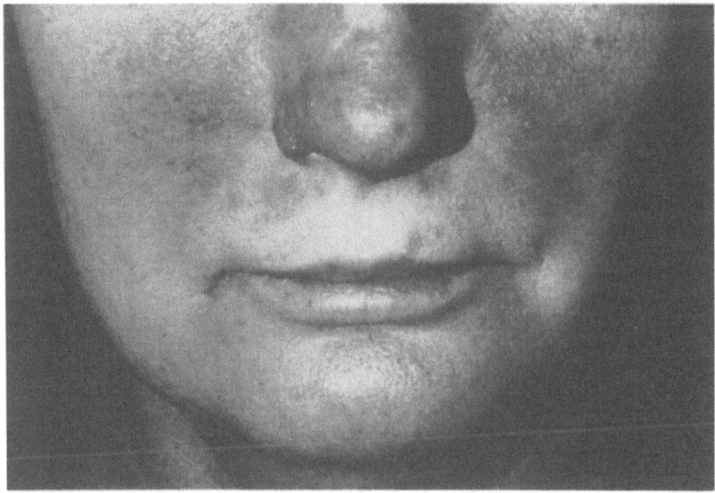

Fig. 11.5 Rosacea papules and pustules.

Fig. 11.6 Jessner's syndrome. (a) Papular lesions affecting the face and trunk, typically affecting the male. (Courtesy of Dr R. S-H. Tan.) (b) Histology of Jessner's syndrome showing dense dermal lymphocytic infiltrate. (Courtesy of Dr T. I. Macleod.)

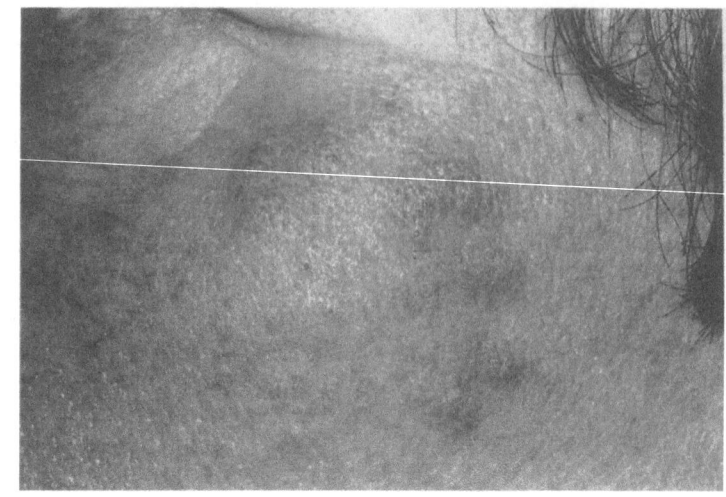

(a)

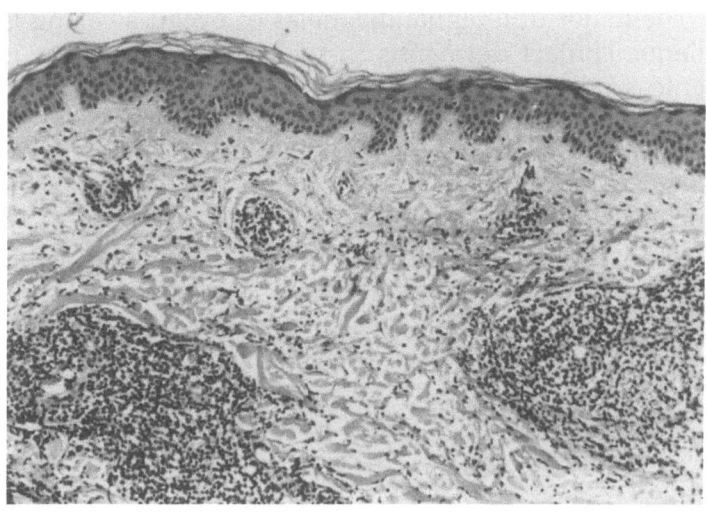

(b)

Fig. 11.7 Seborrhoeic dermatitis of face, showing characteristic scaling on cheek and nasolabial folds. Associated pustulation is common.

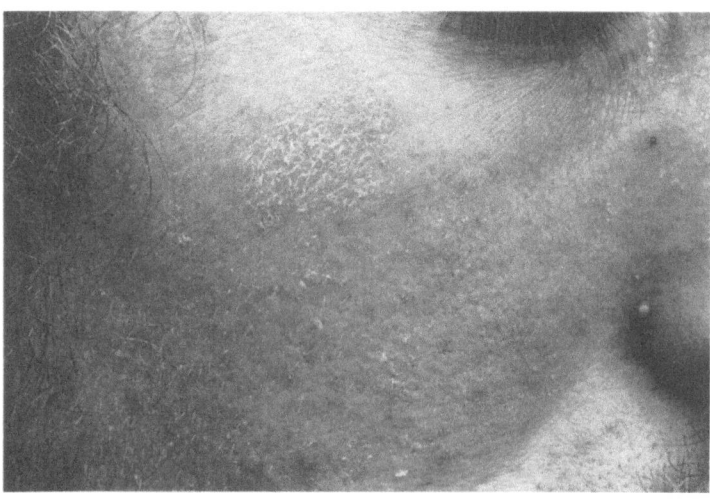

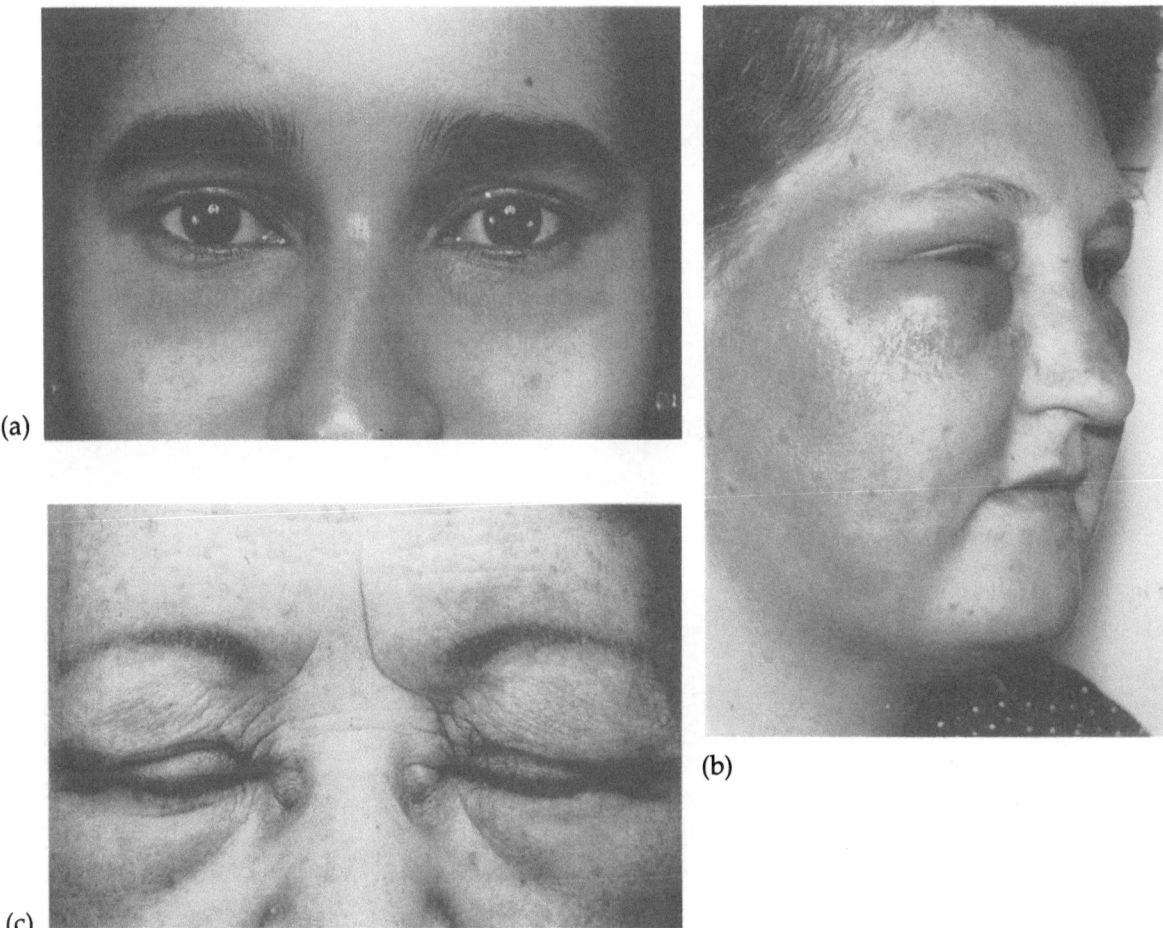

Fig. 11.8 Eyelid swelling. (a) Allergic contact dermatitis due to nail varnish. (b) Erysipelas causing severe oedema of the lower eyelid. (c) Dermatomyositis. Oedema and erythema of upper and lower eyelids.

11.5 MOUTH ULCERS

Aphthous ulcers are painful, well circumscribed, initially pustular becoming punched out with a ragged, sloughing base. They occur frequently in the normal population, but also in such conditions as Behçet's or inflammatory bowel disease.

In Behçet's they tend to be extensive, may also occur in the genital tract and tend to scar. Painless superficial erosions are typically found in Reiter's disease in the oropharynx and may mimic a geographical tongue (Fig.

Fig. 11.9   Geographical tongue in Reiter's disease.

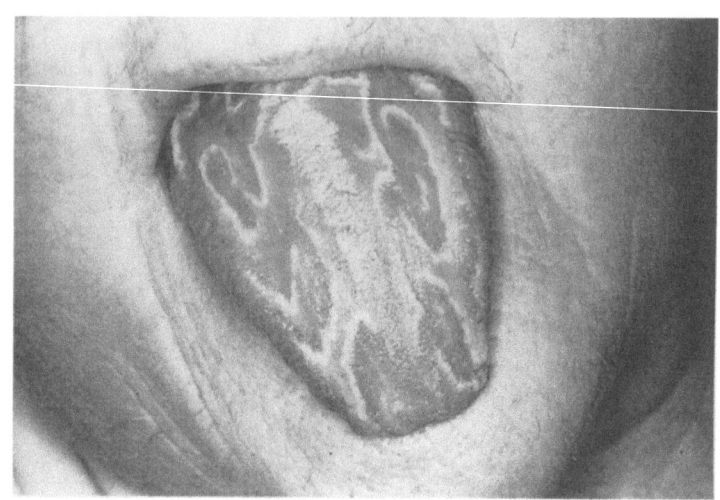

Fig. 11.10   Calcinotic nodule in systemic sclerosis.

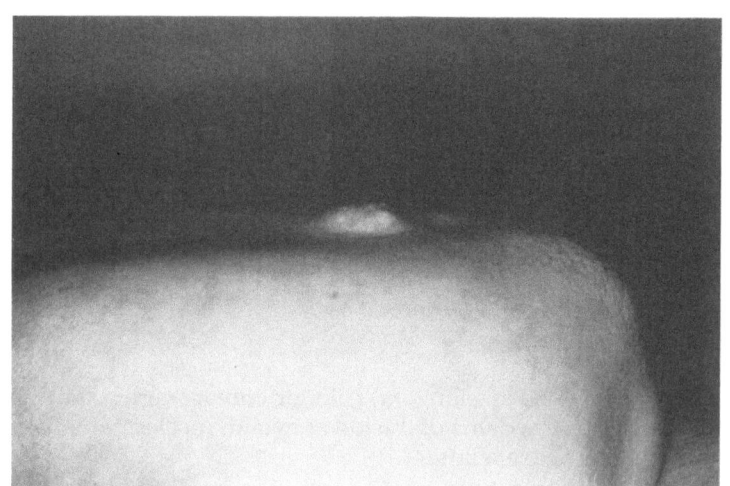

11.9). Painful erosions occur in lupus erythematosus or may be drug induced (see Chapter 10).

11.6   NODULES

Painless nodules can result from granuloma formation, for example, rheumatoid nodules, or deposition of inert material, for example, sodium urate (gouty tophi); or calcium salts, as in systemic sclerosis. They tend to occur at sites of friction and pressure such as the elbow (Fig.

11.10). Painful erythematous nodules associated with joint symptoms are found in erythema nodosum, Sweet's disease and panniculitis (for example, Weber Christian). In generalized nodal osteoarthritis osteophytes developing at the margins of the distal and proximal interphalangeal joints give rise to Heberden's nodes and Bouchard's nodes respectively. In the early phase of their development they may be erythematous and painful (Fig. 11.11).

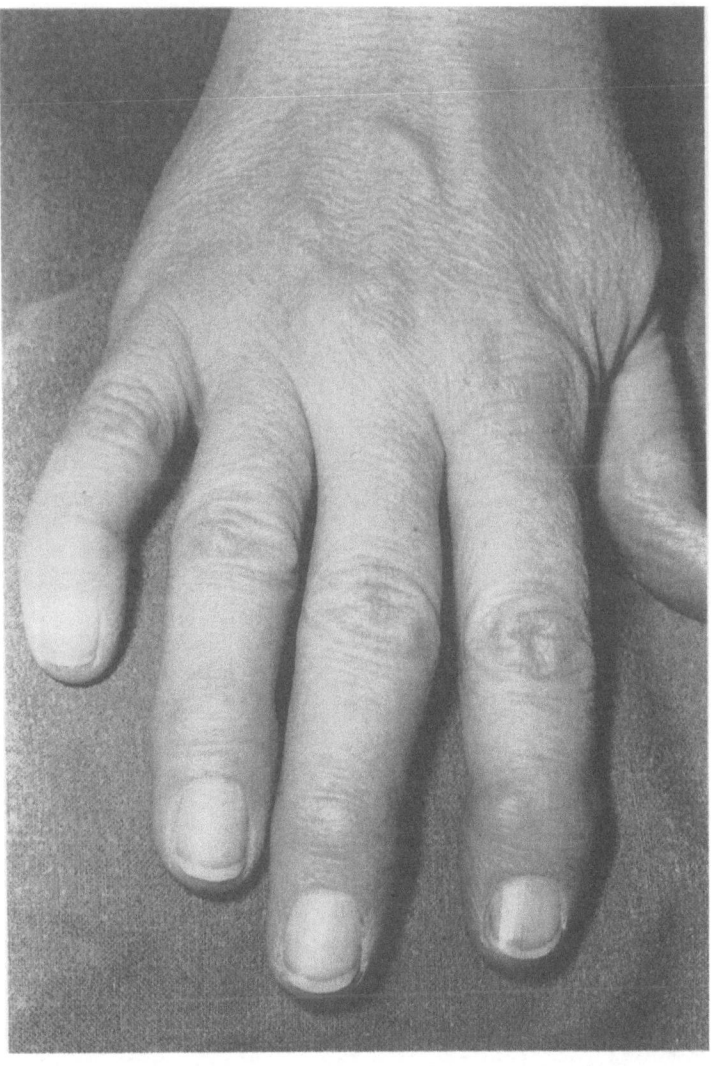

Fig. 11.11 Heberden's nodes affecting the distal interphalangeal joints. Bouchard's nodes similarly affect the proximal interphalangeal joints.

Fig. 11.12 (a) Scarring alopecia in discoid lupus erythematosus. Hyperkeratosis can be found at the base of remaining follicles. Lichen planus may cause indistinguishable changes on the scalp. (b) Scalp involvement in psoriasis ('pityriasis amiantacea'). Hyperkeratosis extends along hair shaft. Scarring is typically absent or minimal. (c) Alopecia areata. Areas of non-scarring alopecia. There may be associated 'exclamation mark' hairs and areas of fine (lanugo) hair regrowth. Eyelids and other hair bearing sites are often involved. Total alopecia may occur and there may be associated nail dystrophy. This may mimic psoriasis, but the pits tend to be larger and shallower and there may also be longitudinal ridging and irregular thickening of the nails.

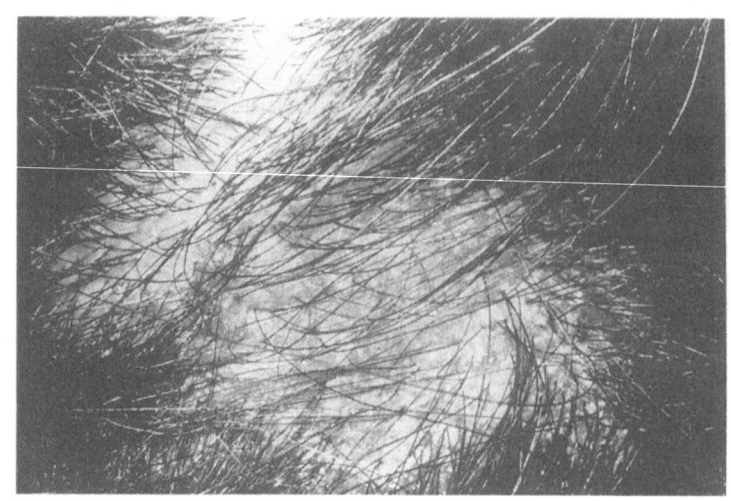

(a)

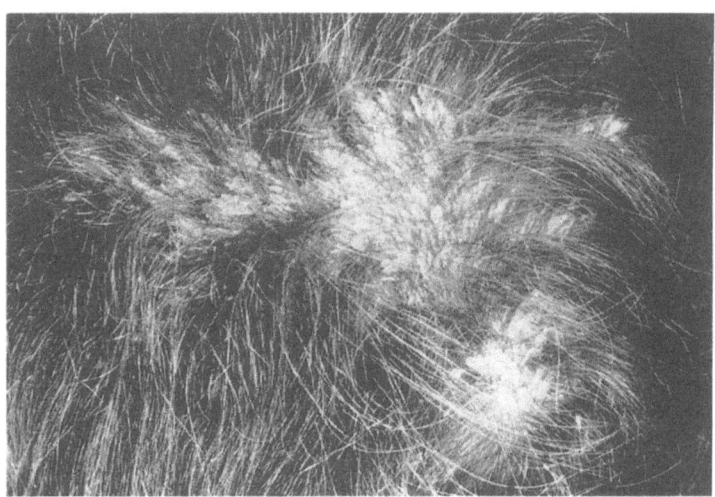

(b)

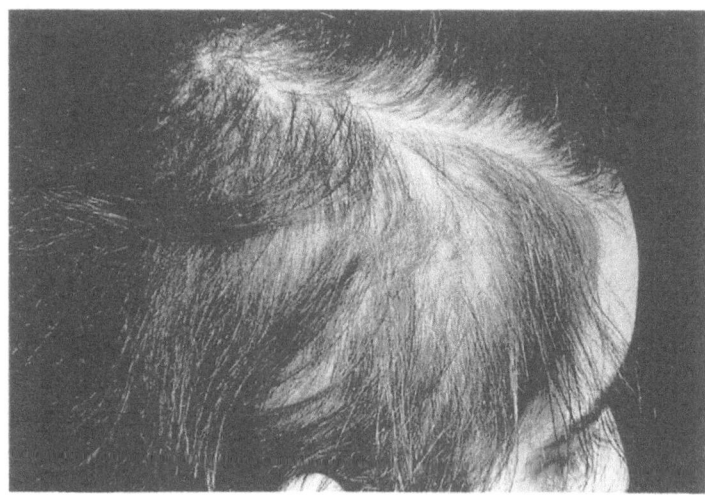

(c)

11.7 ALOPECIA

Diffuse hair loss (up to 80 hairs a day) is a normal process often accentuated at the menopause. However, increasing hair loss may reflect an underlying inflammatory or metabolic disorder such as iron deficiency or thyroid disease. In systemic lupus erythematosus diffuse hair loss reflects disease activity.

Discoid LE and dermatomyositis produce focal scarring alopecia, to be distinguished from alopecia areata and psoriasis (Fig. 11.12).

Index

Page numbers in *italics* refer to figures.

Acetanilide 14
Acne fulminans *120*, 121
Acropachy 105, *107*
Acrosclerosis 18–22
  chronic paronychia in 19, *20*
  contracture of fingers in *19*
  facial appearance in *22*
  ischaemic ulcers in 19, *20*
  pseudoclubbing in 20, *21*
  reduced eversion of eyelid in
    20, *21*
  telangiectasia in 21, *22*
Addison's disease 23
Aldolase 54
Allergic contact dermatitis 51
Allopurinol, side-effects 131
Alopecia
  alopecia areata 89, 143
  diagnosis 142, 143
  non-scarring in systemic LE
    37, *38*, 143
  scarring
    in dermatomyositis 49, 143
    in discoid LE 31, 33, *142*,
      143
Alpha receptor antagonists 25
Anaemia of chronic disease 6
Ankylosing spondylitis 68
Antibiotics 82, 94, 99
Anticentromere antibody
    (ACA) 23
  in CREST 16, *19*
  in systemic sclerosis 13
Antifibrinolytic agents 25
Antimalarials 47, 54
  side-effects 129–30
Antinuclear antibodies 6
Aphthous mucous membrane
    ulceration 79
Arthritis mutilans 72, *73*
Aspirin 122
  side-effects 123
Azathioprine 47, 74, 76
  side-effects 129

Behçet's syndrome 118, 139
  aphthosis in *119*
Benoxaprofen, side-effects 123
Benzalkonium chloride,
    side-effects *131*, 132
Beta-blocker therapy, Raynaud's
    phenomenon and 133
Borellia burgdorferi 97, 99
Bouchard's nodes 141
Bullous morphoea 11

C reactive protein 6
Calcium channel blockers 25
Captopril 26
Carcinomata, as side-effect of
    X-ray therapy 131
Carpal tunnel syndrome 26
Charçot's joints in syphilis 100
Cheiroarthropathy 103, *107*
Chilblain LE 31, 33, *35*
Childhood dermatomyositis 16
  calcinosis universalis in *51*, 5
Chlorambucil, side-effects 129
Chronological sequence of
    disease manifestations
Churg–Strauss syndrome 58,
    60–1, 62
Cinnamates 46
Clofazimine 78
Clutton's joints in syphilis 100
Coal tar 73, 74
Colchicine 26
Cold sensitivity 2
Corticosteroids
  in eosinophilic fasciitis 26
  in lupus erythematosus 47
  in psoriatic arthritis 71, 74
  in rheumatoid arthritis 89, 90,
    91
  in rheumatoid arthritis
    vasculitis 85
  in septic arthritis 92
  side-effects *128*, 129
  see also Steroids

Coup de sabre 10
Creatine phosphokinase (CPK)
    52, 54, 108
CREST syndrome 15, 16–18, 19
Crohn's disease 78
  cheilitis in 79, 81
  fistulae in perianal skin in 79,
    80
CT scanning 7
Cushing's syndrome 52
Cutaneous LE, differential
    diagnosis 43
Cyclophosphamide 47, 90
  side-effects 129
Cyclophosponide, side-effects
    129
Cytomegalovirus (CMV) 100
Cytotoxics, side-effects 129

D-penicillamine 26, 91
  side-effects 123–7
Dapsone 47, 66, 78
Degos' syndrome 38
Dermatomyositis 49–56
  childhood, calcinosis
    universalis in 51, *53*
  clinical features 4, 49–51
  differential diagnosis 51–2
  hyperpigmentation in *50*
  investigations 54
  nail involvement in 49, *52*
  pathogenesis 52–3
  sites of involvement 51
  treatment and prognosis 54
Diabetes 103, 105
  and haemochromatosis 109
  ischaemic ulcers in *107*
Diffuse scleroderma 22–4
Discoid LE 30–4, 45
  prognosis 47
Disease distribution, pattern
    of 1
Distal interphalangeal (DIP)
    joint disease 72

Dithranol 73

Ehlers–Danlos syndrome (EDS) 103, 104
  cigarette paper scarring 103, *105*
Electromyography (EMG) 54
Enteropathic arthropathy 78–82
Eosinophilic fasciitis *25, 26*
Erythema chronicum migrans following tick bite 97, *98*
Erythema marginatum in rheumatic fever *93, 94*
Erythema nodosum 78
  and sarcoidosis 111
  streptococci as cause of 94
Erythema nodosum leprosum 100
Erythema infectiosum 100
Erythrocyte sedimentation rate 6
Essential mixed cryoglobulinaemia in vasculitis 65
Etretinate 74
Eyelid swelling 137, *139*

Facial morphoea *10*
Felty's syndrome 89
Fenbufen, side-effects 123
Finger clubbing in infective endocarditis *97*

Gangrene
  in acrosclerosis 19
  in overlap syndrome 55
  in polyarteritis nodosa *60*
  in systemic lupus erythematosus 38
  in systemic sclerosis 25
Geographical tongue 139, *140*
Giant cell arteritis 66–7
Giant urticaria *121*
Gold, oral 47, 91
  side-effects 128–9
Gonococcal pustules 94, *95*
Gottron's papules 49
Gout 5, 6, 7, 109, 119, *120*
Graft-versus-host (GVH) disease 8
Graves' disease 51, 105
Guttate morphoea 11

Hairy cell leukaemia 58
Heberden's nodes 5, 141
Henoch–Schonlein purpura 65

distribution *64*
  streptococci as cause of 94
Hepatis B surface antigen (HBAg) 57
History-taking 1
Homogentisic acid oxidase 109
Human immunodeficiency virus (HIV) 76, 102
Hydroquinone 109
Hydroxychloroquine 46
  photosensitivity due to 136
Hyperlipidaemia 108–9

Indirect immunofluorescence of CREST 19
Infectious mononucleosis 100
Infective endocarditis 96–7
Inflammatory bowel disease 139
Investigation
  joint disease 6–7
  skin 5–6

Jaccoud's arthropathy 40, 94
Janeway lesions 96
Jejunoileal bypass surgery 79–82
Jessner's lymphocytic infiltrate 34–5, 137, *138*

Kawasaki disease 60
Keratoderma blennorrhagica, *see* Reiter's disease
Kveim test 5

Large vessel vasculitis 38, 57, 66–7
Lassar's Paste 74
Leprosy 100, *101*
Leucocytoclastic vasculitis *63*
Lichen planus due to penicillamine *125*
Lichen sclerosus et atrophicus 9, 12
Light sensitivity, *see* Photosensitivity
Linear localized scleroderma 11–13
Linear morphoea *10*, 11–13
  evolution of cutaneous involvement in 14–15
  treatment 13
Livedo reticularis *59, 60*
Lupus band test 44
Lupus crisis 40
Lupus erythematosus (LE) 26–48

aetiology and pathogenesis 27–9
diagnosis 41–4
direct immunofluorescence in 5
drug-induced 28, 29
general clinical features 4, 30
histology 29–30
serology 45–6
spectrum of 27
Lupus erythematosus profundus (panniculitis) 31, *36*
Lupus nephritis 29
Lupus pernio 114
Lupus vulgaris 33
Lyme disease 97–9

Marfan's syndrome 103
Mepacrine 46
  side-effects 130
Methamphetamine abuse 58
Methotrexate 54, 74, 77, 83, 90
Minocycline 78
Morphoea 8–13
  generalized 8–11, 24
  plaque 8
MRI 7
Mucocutaneous lymph node syndrome 60
Multicentric reticulohistiocytosis 115–17
  bone resorption in *118*
Myasthenia gravis 41
Mycobacterium leprae 100

Necrotizing vasculitis 57, 58–63
  histology 58
  prognosis and treatment of 62–3
Neisseria infection 94–6
Neisseria meningitidis 95–6
Neonatal lupus erythematosus 41, *42*
Nitroglycerine 25
Nodules 140–1
Non-steroidal anti-inflammatory drugs (NSAIDs)
  in aphthous mucous membrane ulceration 79
  in erythema nodosum 78
  in jejunoileal bypass surgery 80
  in lupus erythematosus 47
  photosensitivity due to 136

in psoriatic arthritis 74
in Reiter's syndrome 76
side-effects 123, 134

Ochronosis 109, *110*
Onycholysis 133, 134
in psoriasis 71
Osteogenesis imperfecta 103
Otitis media 58
Overlap syndromes 50, 55–6
Oxyphenbutazone, side-effects 123

Panniculitis (LE profundus) 31, *36*
Papular LE 34–6
Para-aminobenzoic acid 46
Pemphigoid as side-effect 125, *126*
Pemphigus erythematosus (Senear-Usher syndrome) 35
Pemphigus foliaceus due to penicillamine 126, *127*
Pemphigus vulgaris due to penicillamine *126, 127*
Penicillamine 13
side-effects 125–7
Penicillin 58
Phenylbutazone 58
Phenytoin in linear morphoea 13
Photo-onycholysis *134*
Photosensitivity 1, 3, 123, 136
Physical examination 2–5
joints 4–5
skin 2–4
Pityriasis amiantacea 142
Plaque morphoea 8
Polyarteritis nodosa (PAN) 57, 58, 59–60, 87
gangrene and haemorrhagic bullae due to *60*
livedo reticularis in *59*, 60
punched out necrotic ulcers in *59*, 60
Polychrondritis 58
Polymyalgia rheumatica (PMR) 52
Polymyositis 7
Porphyria cutanea tarda 41
Prednisolone 54
Prostacyclin 25
Prostaglandin El 25
Pseudoclubbing 20, *21*
Pseudoxanthoma elasticum

(PXE) 103, *106*
Psoriasis
diagnosis 3
disease distribution 1
family history 2
psoriatic arthritis 69–74
joints in 5, *73*
nail involvement *71*
psoriatic plaque *69*, 70
Psoriatic onycholysis 134
Pustular psoriasis *70*
PUVA 77
Pyoderma gangrenosum 78, *79*, 88

Radioisotope imaging 7
Rapeseed oil as cause of systemic sclerosis 13–14
Raynaud's phenomenon
in acrosclerosis 19
cold sensitivity 2
in dermatomyositis 50
diagnosis 133–5
in diffuse scleroderma 23
distinction from generalized morphoea 11
in large vessel arteritis 66
in overlap syndromes 55
in rheumatoid arthritis 89
in systemic lupus erythematosus 39
in systemic sclerosis 14, 15
treatment for 25
ulceration 3
vinyl chloride as cause of 14
Reiter's syndrome 72, 74–7
Achilles tendinitis in 5
association with HIV virus 102
circinate balanitis in *75*
course and prognosis 77
keratoderma blenorrhagica in *76*
management 76–7
mouth ulcers in 139
'red eye' in *75*, 77
sacroiliitis in *77*
Retinoids, systemic 77
Retroviruses and LE 28
Rheumatic fever 5, 94
Rheumatoid arthritis 58, 59
confusion with CREST syndrome 16
cutaneous ulceration 87–8, 90
drug treatment in 1
hand joints in *4, 5*

hyperpigmentation in *90*
joint rupture 88–9
management 90–1
palmar erythema in *89*
rheumatoid factor 6
rheumatoid nodules 83–5
septic arthritis 90
skin in 82–91
in systemic sclerosis 24
vasculitis 85–7
Rheumatoid factor 6
RNA polymerase 1 in systemic sclerosis 13
Rosacea papules, diagnosis 137
Rowell's syndrome 37
Rubella 100–2

Saddle-nose deformity
in syphilis 100
in Wegener's syndrome 56
Salazopyrin (sulphasalazine) 13
side-effects 129, *130*
Sarcoid dactylitis *115, 116*
Sarcoidosis 111–15
giant cells in *116*, 117
Kveim test in 5
lupus pernio in *114*, 115
sarcoid dactylitis in *115, 116*
sarcoid nodules 112, *114*
xanthelasma palpebrarum in *116, 117*
Sausage digits 5, 39, 55, 72
Scalp examination 3
Sclerodactyly 15
Scleroderma 8–26
causes 11
Scleroderma of Buschke 25
Scurvy 110
perifollicular haemorrhages in *111*
Seborrheic dermatitis 137, *138*
Senear–Usher syndrome 35
Septic arthritis 5, 92–4
Sjogren's syndrome 21, 41, 46, 89
Skin lesions 1–2
Small vessel vasculitis 37, 57, 63–6
Small cell vasculitis, treatment 65–6
Spanish oil disease 14
Spirochaetal infections 97–100
Splinter haemorrhages in infective endocarditis 96, *97*

Staphylococcal infections 90, 92
Steroids
  in dermatomyositis 54
  in giant cell arteritis 67
  in lupus erythematosus 47
  in plaque morphoea 13
  in pyoderma gangrenosum 78
  in Reiter's disease 77
  in Takayasu's disease 66
Still's disease 111, *112*
Streptococcal infections, beta-
      haemolytic 64, 94
Subacute cutaneous LE 36–7, 45
Subcutaneous morphoea 11
Sulphasalazine
      (salazopyrin) 76, 79
Sulphonamides 58, 64
  side-effects, 129, 130
Sun protection factor 46
Sweet's syndrome (acute
      neutrophilic
      dermatosis) 18, 141
Syphilis, papules in *99*, 100
Systemic lupus erythematosus
      (SLE) 37–41
  antinuclear antibodies in 6–7
  ARA criteria for 43
  arthritis in *40*
  butterfly erythema in 37, *38*
  clinical features 30
  clinical manifestations of 38
  distinction from
      dermatomyositis 51
  features characterizing 44
  genetics of 27
  immunological abnormalities
      29

photosensitivity 28
prognosis 47
serological findings in 45
treatment 46–7
vasculitic lesions in *39*
Systemic sclerosis 13–26
  antibodies in 46
  coexistence with linear
      morphoea 11–12
  cutaneous involvement 14, *15*
  differential diagnosis 24–5
  distinction from generalized
      morphoea 8
  joint involvement in *23*
  toxins causing 13, 14
  treatment 25–6
Takayasu's disease 66
Tetracyclines 77
  side-effects *134*
Thalidomide 47
Thiazides 58, 64
Thyotoxicosis 72
Thyroid disease 105–8
Tick bite 97, *98*
Titanium dioxide 46
Topoisomerase 1, 24
Toxoplasma 52
Treponema pallidum 99–100
Tuberculoid leprosy 34
Tuberculous synovitis 7
Spondyloarthropathies 68–82
  definition 68–9

Ulcerative colitis (UC) 78
Ulcers
  in acrosclerosis 19, *20*

aphthous mucous
      membrane 79
  in CREST 19–20
  in diabetes *107*
  digitial 2, 3, 25
  mouth 2, 139–40
  orogenital 2
  punched out necrotic *59*, *60*,
      88
  in pyoderma gangrenosum *79*
  in Raynaud's phenomenon 3
  in rheumatoid arthritis 87–8
  in syphilis 100
  urticaria 122
  giant *121*

Vasculitis 7, 57–67
  classification 57
Verrucous LE 31, 34
Vibration white finger 133
Villonodular synovitis 7
Vinyl chloride as cause of
      systemic sclerosis 14
Viral infections 64, 100–2
Vitiligo in rheumatoid arthritis
      89

Weber Christian
      panniculitis 141
Wegener's syndrome 58, 62
  pathological features *61*
  saddle-nose deformity *62*
Wickham's striae *125*

Xanthelasmata 116, *117*

Zinc oxide 46